The Youth Plan

Look Younger. Feel Great. Here's How.

First published in Great Britain in 2018 on behalf of:
Rejuvenated Ltd
Tel: (+44) 1142 356 585
Email: info@rejuvenated.co.uk
www.rejuvenated.com

Published by:
RMC Media – www.rmcmedia.co.uk
6 Broadfield Court, Sheffield, S8 0XF
Tel: 0114 250 6300

Author: Kathryn Danzey
Design: Dan Wray
Proof-reader: Christopher Brierley

Printed and bound in Malta by:
Gutenberg Press Ltd – www.gutenberg.com.mt
Gudja Road, Tarxien, Malta, GXQ 2902
Tel: 00356 2189 7037

A CIP catalogue record for this book is available from the British Library.

ISBN: 978-1-907998-35-5

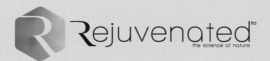

FEED YOUR INNER BEAUTY

INTRODUCTION

Do you want the secret to beautiful, brighter, glowing skin? To understand how to enjoy bags of energy and vitality? And to live a healthier, happier life?

If you answered 'yes' to any of those questions – and I'm guessing that you did! – then you've come to the right place. The Rejuvenated Lifestyle has been designed just for you, and can help to transform your life.

While it may sound too good to be true, I promise that it's not! By curling up and reading on, you can discover how you can have:

- **Glowing, hydrated skin – at any age**
- **Healthy, balanced blood sugar levels**
- **More vitality and soaring energy levels**
- **A lean, strong body**
- **A redefined body shape – for life**

As well as this, the Rejuvenated way of life will help to keep you on track with eating healthily, making it as simple and as enjoyable as possible.

With our guidance, you can embrace a whole new approach to eating. There will be:

- **No points**
- **No sins**
- **No counting**

We simply want you to turn to nourishing and delicious whole foods. Pure, natural and honest.

Are you ready to join in the Rejuvenated revolution? Read on...

Shine From The Inside, Out:

If you ever sneak a peek in the mirror when you wake in the morning and dislike what you see, then you're not alone. In fact, I think we've all been there, feeling frustrated or upset at our own reflections.

Yet, it doesn't have to be that way – it is possible to feel beautiful and youthful, no matter what your age. Whether your skin looks or feels tired, dull, dehydrated, or refuses to glow no matter what lotions and potions you apply, then this book is for you.

Over the last 40 years, I've dedicated my career to discovering some truly life-changing things that can make a huge difference to your health, and to how you look and feel.

We all want to look and feel great but, let's be honest, we don't always think about our long-term health. Yet, the Rejuvenated life will start to change that, step by little step. As you read on, try to see this as your beauty bible; your go-to book to help you feel amazing right now, and in the future.

I want to share how you can look and feel amazing – right now – and how to combine with all the benefits of health and longevity. It might sound like a mountain to climb, but I promise that we will get there, and it's easier than you may think. Together, we can – and will - do this.

In the Western world, medical advances mean we're all living longer, but that's not the only thing that matters – the quality of health we enjoy should be important, too.

For me, the key is in having life in your years, rather than simply years in your life. Both of my parents died at 67. They were young in spirit and seemed healthy, but my father died of a heart attack and my mother spent her last ten years battling cancer. It is this that has spurred me on, and I am driven to find answers for both my family and for you.

Of course, as you read on, you'll find that some of these tips will fit into your life, while some of them won't. Sometimes you'll be on it, and sometimes you won't (let's face it, we all have "off" days!). But, if you sprinkle a few Rejuvenated principles into your regime, you'll soon find you have more energy and a real zest for life. Not only will you feel brighter, but you'll soon be shining from the inside, out.

A FULL-CIRCLE APPROACH

Now, enjoying a healthier, happier and more vibrant life may mean some changes.

Yet, how hard can it be to move a bit more, to give sugars a swerve and to drink more water? It's easy, really, when you think about it – it's just that so many other things, our lives really, get in the way.

I'm no different to you; I find it as easy as anyone else to go off track. Take last year, when I had to stare a few of my own demons in the eye when my eldest got married.

One of the things I hate is having my photo taken. Yet, as mothers-of-the-bride or groom know all too well, these photos hang from the walls forever, and there's no avoiding the camera or simply cowering in the corner! At 60 I really wanted to look and feel my best. I knew what I should do, and I'm pretty healthy generally, but this meant extra action.

The fact is, nutrition and diet are only part of the solution. For us to be at our best, and to stay there, we need to combine it with positive changes to our lifestyle. Regular exercise, peace of mind, and general well-being all play their part, too, yet I bet that many of you will find at least one of these a little tricky – my weaknesses are committing to regular exercise and to de-stressing.

As the wedding slowly crept upon us, I knew that I had to make changes. Nothing drastic, but I decided to exercise every day and to meditate, too. I also made a few tweaks to my diet, and was thrilled to find that my body transformed.

Happily, not only has the weight that I lost stayed off, but the body transformation has stayed with me, too. The changes I made became game-changers in longevity and health – all along, Rejuvenated was the answer.

If that sounds out-of-reach, then I promise it's not – you can do it too, and this book will share how to.

I'll be with you, every step of the way, guiding you along to help you be in your best ever health and shape. Together, we will feel fantastic again and, at the end of those four weeks, you'll be shining from the inside, out.

...and don't worry how you might get on after the next four weeks because you can now log into all our special tips and advice at www.rejuvenated.com. We are going to support and guide you ongoing, that way you will be able stay feeling just amazing

Want to join me? Read on to reveal my favourite tips to help you to unveil your inner beauty, to keep you feeling at your best, and to live a longer, healthier Rejuvenated life.

WHO AM I?

Of course, what use is our journey together if you don't know who I am, and how I can help?

So let's get started.

My name is Kathryn, and I've worked in the health and beauty industry for a long time now – over 40 years, in fact. I've picked up all sorts of wonders and miracles along the way. The decisive breakthrough came 25 years ago when I started to connect nutrition to the treatments we used in our clinic.

As soon as I made that connection, I quickly realised the incredible benefit of eating healthily – the difference we saw when we combined good nutrition with great skincare was staggering.

As a result, we started offering clients nutritional programmes to use alongside their skincare routine and treatments. The results were amazing, and those who embraced it would return the following month, saying they had more vitality. Not only this, but they said that they were 'shining from the inside, out'.

The more I looked into nutrition, the more incredible it seemed to me that skincare brands added extracts of ingredients, such as grapes and papaya, into their products. These are all antioxidants which protect the skin but to me it made sense to eat these potent extracts and see far superior benefits? And not just for the face, but the whole body, too!

Eventually my passion led to us sitting down and chatting to an elite sports nutrition company. We got on brilliantly, and developed a relationship with a team who were also interested in challenging the concepts of conventional nutrition. We bantered about theories on hydration and the healing of tissues – all super geeky things, but fascinating to me, nonetheless!

I became excited, and quickly I started thinking that if you could work wonders on athletes, then you could do the same for us normal folk, too. In fact, I truly believe that the right products and nutrition can see endless benefits for the health and wellbeing of both an individual and their skin.

Together, we discovered the perfect blend of sporting, nutritional excellence and powerful, natural ingredients – and the answer I'd been searching for all along.

However, not everyone thought the same way, and so we came up against a few walls. We quickly discovered that, while eating healthily was the best way to protect our well-being, most people were only interested in health when they become ill. Then, they take care of themselves until they are better, before going back to existing habits.

It set me thinking towards creating a simple solution: having a drink to make you look younger was an incredible, yet easy, way for people to think about their ongoing health, every single day. Eventually, the concept of beauty from within helped us to influence a healthier and more Rejuvenated Lifestyle.

By 2010, we launched the first collagen drink on the market. We were so far ahead of the game that we were leading the way, paving the way for others to follow. The incredible relationship that we created with our development team means we have a whole series of new products planned for the next five years.

Of course, the beauty and health industry constantly changes and evolves. The scientifically-proven treatments are always improving, while the food we ate just ten years ago is very different to what we eat now. Our lifestyles are ever-changing, too, yet there are some constants that we should all embrace as the cornerstone of our programme for health.

These are the cornerstones that I want to share in this book...

DITCH THE DIETS

No matter how much you try to lift and smooth every fine line and wrinkle, your skin will still look tired and sallow if you don't nourish it from within.

It's probably taken over half a century, but we are now slowly starting to realise that diets simply don't work. On a diet, you might shed the pounds at first, but then they gradually pile back on.

If that sounds all too familiar, then don't worry – we have the answers. With Rejuvenated, you can break that cycle, enjoy radiant vitality, find your inner balance and shine from the inside, out.

As you know, I've been where you possibly are now. Yet, after years of trying different diets – some faddy, many impossible to stick to – I found that by simply eating healthily, my body was completely transformed. My skin was vibrant, my energy levels soared, and those niggling aches and pains disappeared altogether.

My lesson? Well, it's simple, really! Diets are not the answer, and they never have been. The key is to enjoy a healthier, happier lifestyle, and you will soon reap the rewards.

It's also important to stop being too hard on yourself, and to remember that we're all individuals. We have different lifestyles, genes and environments, and what works for someone else might not be quite right for you. This book takes that into account and gives you the guidelines to work from so that you can create your own plan for your future health and wellbeing.

Are you with me?

I hope so! The information in this book will help you to reveal the brand new, Rejuvenated you.

HOW TO USE REJUVENATED

Now that you're part of the Rejuvenated revolution, how do you use this book to achieve the best possible results? Well, read on!

In the first half of the book, you'll find the information you need to help you to make the best choices for your health and wellbeing. You'll understand what you should avoid, and you'll also be empowered with the knowledge to switch on your youth factor.

The second half of the book has a four-week healthy eating plan to set you on your way. This includes menus, a food diary and shopping lists. If you're feeling eager and want to start straight away, then you can always skip straight to this section!

Are you ready to join me? Let the magic begin...

'Let food be thy medicine and medicine be thy food'

When you have a moment, I'd like you to stop and think about this quote from the ancient Greek physician Hippocrates.

More than 2,000 years since he first uttered those famous words, and it still rings true – and it's exactly what the Rejuvenated revolution is based upon.

All those years ago, Hippocrates was believed to have been the founder of modern medicine, or medicine as we now know it. Way ahead of his time, he made the connection that the body needs to be treated as a whole, rather than looking at individual niggles or symptoms.

As the health pioneer of his age, Hippocrates looked at the way our lives could affect our bodies. He believed that everything was connected, that our food, environment, exercise, even the seasons and where we live could change our health, for better or for worse.

Fast forward through the centuries, and you'll find that things are a little different now. Each culture has discovered its own healing traditions and medical marvels. Yet, as science became more and more advanced with some truly incredible discoveries, many of these ancient traditions became lost.

Don't get me wrong, there are now many wondrous and life-changing medicines that we simply could not live without. Yet, today's medicine often focuses on specific diseases, without necessarily looking for the root cause of an illness, or why we may be feeling this way.

The key is to bring everything together, to use all the tools we have, right at our fingertips. Together, modern medicine and our lifestyle are formidable allies, and they give us all the tools we need in our quest for longevity and youth.

Throughout Rejuvenated, I'll be sharing with you how your health is interlinked with not only your food choices, but also your stress levels, your choice of career and fitness levels, and even the relationships in your life.

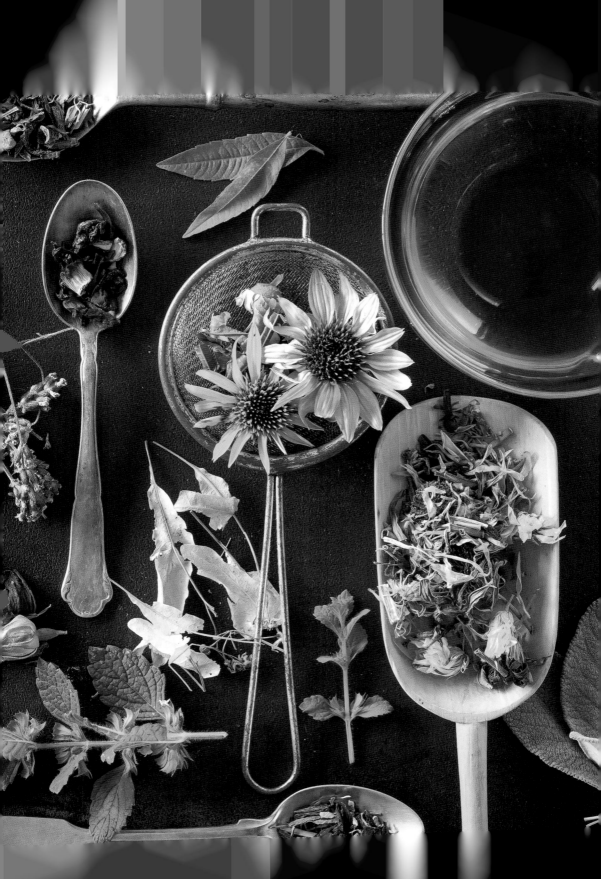

FOODS FOR YOUTHFULNESS

Is it possible to turn back the ageing clock?

Do you ever look in the mirror and wonder where the years have gone? I'm guessing that this is true for many of us – and you may be wondering what you can do.

Of course, however much we may want to, we can't change our chronological age, or the number of years that we've been on the planet for. However, we can appear more youthful and wind back the years by having vitality, youthfulness and gorgeous, glowing skin.

Our biological age shows how our bodies are wearing, and is a truer measure of your health rather than those ticking years. Our lifestyles can play a big part in determining this – making good choices can wind back the clock, while poor lifestyles may see us age beyond our years.

This means that you don't have to look your age – you can be as young as you feel, or as young as you want to feel!

This book will share how you can remove your mirror image; how you can be more beautiful and simply glow.

While it may sound unrealistic, I promise that it isn't.

As science starts to make huge strides in discovering the elements that can protect our cells and DNA to help maintain a youthful look. You might not be able to change your actual age, but you can re-set your biological age – and this book will show you how.

How can you take years off your biological age?

It isn't just about the foods you eat, although that is a large part of it. There are other key and important elements that can add or take away those years.

First of all, poor decisions in our lifestyle produce harmful responses at a cellular level and, in turn, create inflammation in the body. When our bodies are constantly inflamed, even at a low level, this stimulates an autoimmune response and can cause the immune system to start attacking healthy tissue. This can eventually cause diseases such as asthma, arthritis, type II diabetes, peptic ulcers and bowel disease. It can even block our ability to burn fat.

Yet, what many of us don't realise is that we can change much of this. For instance, we can challenge our body's ability to burn fat. Yes, you read that right – we can change the way our bodies burn fat, if only you know how!

The thing is, the body has a small amount of brown, fat-burning cells, which are hidden mostly in our shoulders and neck. These amazing cells burn fat far more effectively and efficiently than the more common white fat cells.

The problem is, many of us who struggle with our weight have just a handful of these brown cells, which can lie fairly dormant. However, it is possible to change this, and we can convert white fat to brown fat cells by exercising or by exposing ourselves to freezing cold temperatures.

I understand that this in itself can be something of an uphill battle! Particularly when many of us are leading more and more sedentary lifestyles and live in cosy, central-heated homes. This makes stimulating the production of these all-important brown fat cells a far more difficult task.

What's more, this is made worse as inflammation directly interferes with the signals that create this process. Yet, don't despair! Certain ingredients and foods can help, and I'll talk about those later.

In the meantime, simply replacing inflammatory-causing patterns with healthy ones can tip the scales in your favour – we can turn down inflammation and turn on youthfulness. No matter how old you are or how you feel at this moment, you can improve your biological age.

I'm in my 60th year, but my biological clock is much younger – and I promise that yours can be, too. The secret to being your most youthful, no matter what your age, is this:

- **Thought for food**
- **Taking key supplements**
- **Super hydration**
- **Exercise**
- **Relaxation and sleep**

Now, let's delve a little deeper and explore each of these on its own...

WEEK 1

Supercharged Foods For A Strong Body

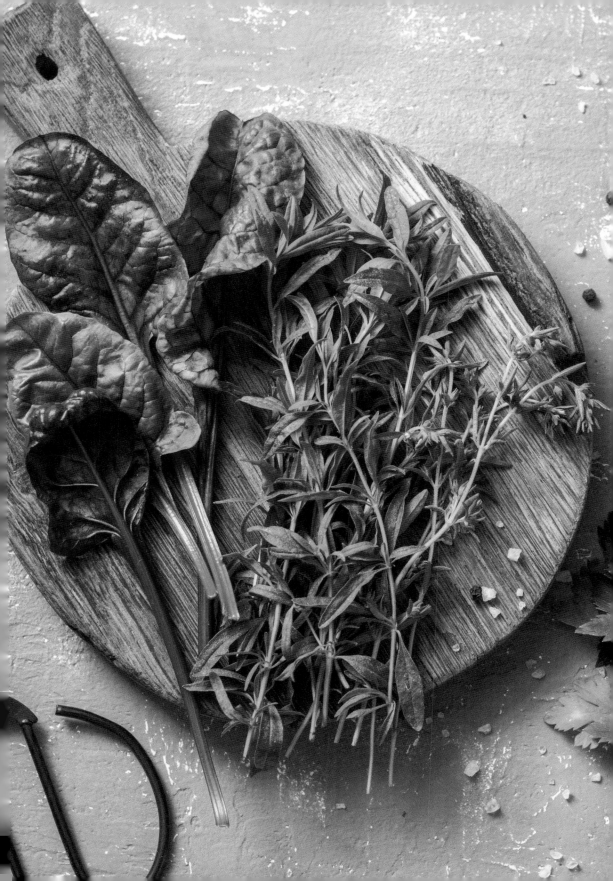

Thought for Food

In the first week of your new, Rejuvenated Lifestyle, we'll be looking at the foods that can switch on youth, and ditching the ones which add to the aches in your body and the lines on your face.

An inflammatory diet is one full of fried foods, fizzy drinks, too much caffeine, sugars and pre-packaged products. However tempting they may seem, eating too many of these foods can trigger a level of inflammation which prevents cells from functioning correctly.

On the flipside, loading your plates with foods rich in antioxidants, minerals and good fats will nourish your cells. Think of natural, fresh foods that cover the whole spectrum of the rainbow.

I have to admit that, for me, the best way to avoid the inflammatory foods was to simply take a bin liner and ditch the rubbish. It's a little bit harsh but take a good, hard look at what you have in your fridge and cupboards. Plan your next shopping trip to avoid 'empty', processed foods and restock with beautiful rainbows of nutrient-dense produce for health and vitality. You'll find our four week eating plan comes with shopping lists to make this so much easier.

You'll quickly notice a difference, too – and it will get easier by the day. In fact, you'll soon find that when you start your morning with health-giving foods, you'll want to eat even less of those nutritionally-devoid foods.

So, let's delve some more. Which foods should you be avoiding to delay ageing and inflammation, and which should you be adding to your plates?

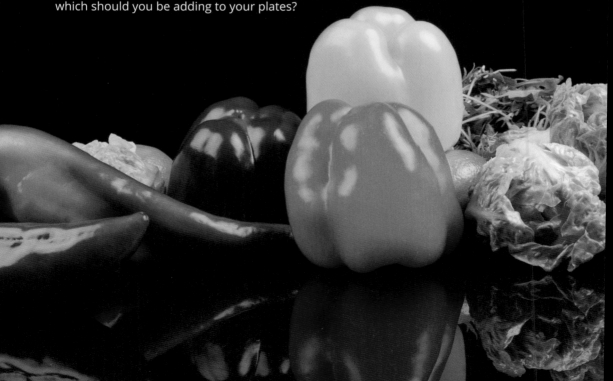

1. WHITE CARBS

First up, the obvious culprit: processed carbs. Many of you will probably know that there are two types of sugar – naturally-occurring sugars, like those found in fruit, and refined sugars, such as table sugar. Over recent years, the s-word has become the enemy of the dieting world, with government departments and nutritionists across the globe urging us to kick the habit.

While it seems easier to swear off all sugars, the problem lies with refined sugars and carbohydrates. Think pastries and cakes, bags of white pasta and bread, and the bumper bags of sweets. Eating too many of these can spike our blood sugar levels which, in turn, can trigger all sorts of problems.

A sugar rollercoaster like this can soon take its toll, causing our bodies to go into a meltdown. Eventually, we can become so sensitive to shifts in blood sugar that we release excess insulin. This can then lead to insulin resistance, and, potentially, type II diabetes, obesity and poor immunity.

You probably don't need me to tell you that sugar is also incredibly addictive – the more we eat, the more we want. Scarily, it's actually many times more addictive than cocaine. However, later on I'll share with you the secrets to defeating the cravings that would normally bring on the nibbles.

Yet, before you swear off sugar altogether, please remember this: not all sugars are bad for us. There are those, such as the ones found in fruits and wholemeal foods, that are good for us. While these foods do contain a fair amount of sugar, they're also rich in fibre, which slows down their absorption into the body. They also have great benefits and contain antioxidants, vitamins and minerals that are crucial to our health.

2. FATS: THE GOOD, THE BAD AND THE UGLY

Contrary to decades of dieting advice, recent studies have shown that fats are not the main culprit in obesity. In fact, we need to eat fat to lose fat.

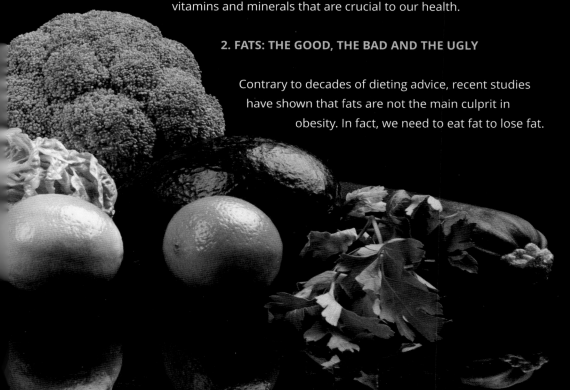

Over the last few years, there's been a huge shift from the 'low-fat' mantra. The truth is, our body needs fats and can't live without them – they form a vital part of our diet. Of course, this doesn't give you free reign to go and eat greasy, fatty foods. We still shouldn't be eating just any old type of fat, nor should we consume it by the bucketload – it's all about moderation, and making the right choices.

The easiest way to do this is to cook from scratch. Before you start panicking, though, don't worry! It doesn't have to take hours to prepare healthy, nutritious foods. Flick to the back of the book, and you'll see that our recipes are quick and easy to make.

It also helps to load up your shopping trolleys with individual foods rather than pre-prepared products. If you do buy manufactured foods, then make sure that you avoid those with 'hydrogenated fat' on the labels. Hydrogenated fats are created by forcing hydrogen into the fat molecules of food, which makes them unnatural and damaging to our health.

Instead, search out unsaturated fats and mono and polyunsaturated fats, which reduce inflammation in the body. The best sources of these fats are from vegetables such as olive, canola, grape seed and other foods such as avocado, coconut, nuts, seeds and fish.

3. DAIRY

This one is a little more tricky – even dieticians can't quite agree on whether or not dairy is good for us. On the one hand, there are those who find it suits their diet perfectly, while others find it inflammatory.

There are also those who are lactose intolerant, while others react to casein, a protein that has a similar structure to whey. Symptoms can range from headaches, congestion, fatigue, bloating and gas to systemic inflammation, including acne. The problem is, the actual process of pasteurisation makes milk harder to digest.

If you do suffer from headaches and bloating, the best way to find out whether or not you can tolerate dairy is to simply go without for a couple of weeks and see how you feel. I personally find that I am less congested and have less bloating, but I do still enjoy the odd cup of tea with milk.

You'll see when you get to our recipe section that we've included some delicious meals with goat's cheese in them, as this can be easier to digest. If you do cut back on dairy and are worried about getting enough calcium in your diet, then chat through things with your doctor or a nutritional advisor. It's worth remembering, though, that almonds, kale, collard greens and spinach are all rich in calcium.

4. GRAINS

Some of us find that wheat, barley and rye can cause inflammation in the body.

There are very few people who are actually allergic to gluten and have the potentially life-threatening autoimmune condition coeliac disease. However, there are a growing number of us who suffer from bowel-related inflammatory conditions, such as IBS (irritable bowel syndrome), which can be triggered by grains.

Scientists are now working on the theory that proteins within these grains may lead to some of us developing non-coeliac gluten sensitivity. One group of proteins found within wheat – amylase-trypsin inhibitors (ATIS) – has been linked to inflammation, which can then spread to other tissues in the body.

Researchers now think it's possible that these proteins can even worsen the symptoms of chronic diseases such as asthma, arthritis, heart disease and multiple sclerosis.

By now, you've probably noticed that the free–from aisles in our supermarkets are growing ever bigger. From gluten-free pizzas to snacks, biscuits and bread, there are all sorts of options out there to suit the growing number of us who are going gluten-free.

However, try to steer clear of these specially-made gluten-free products – many of them are not as healthy as they may seem. Instead, if you feel you'd like to try a gluten-free diet, then cut out all grains for three weeks, rather than buying free-from products. After the three weeks is up, reintroduce these foods, one grain at a time, back into your diet. Try it for two days to see if you notice any bloating or headaches.

5. ALCOHOL

While we know not to go crazy and binge drink, many of us will have heard about how small amounts of alcohol (or, at least, certain kinds!) are good for us. Yet, while the odd glass of red wine can help to protect our heart, I'm sorry to break it to you – alcohol definitely plays a part in weight gain. And that's not just because of the empty calories; alcohol stimulates the release of fat-storing hormones into the blood stream, too.

The problem is, what we see as a couple of cheeky wines can actually overload the liver, meaning it can't get on with the important job of processing fat. As a result, the body switches to fat storing, and the area it favours most is our waistline.

Why does my skin get red when I drink?

Alcohol doesn't just affect the way your favourite jeans do up – it can also ruin the glow you've worked so hard for! A few drinks can dilate the blood vessels, which is why you often feel quite warm and flushed when you drink. Because of this, long-term, regular drinking can cause broken capillaries and leave you with a constant flush.

If you're worried about this, then taking up the Rejuvenated plan will help to calm this down. You can also find lots of tips on our web page www.rejuvenated.com to help reduce skin problems.

Which Are The Rejuvenated Superfoods For Amazing Skin And Health?

Nature has given us an abundance of amazing fruits, vegetables, nuts and pulses to promote health, and beautiful skin is a reflection of this. These foods may be relatively simple, at least in terms of their packaging, yet they actually contain all sorts of goodness, including antioxidants, vitamins, minerals and fibre.

However, before we delve a little further, I want you to try to remember this important piece of advice: when it comes to our diet and our lifestyles, there is no one size fits all, and there is no one food that may work wonders.

We're all individuals, and what suits one person may not suit you. If you feel unsure, try to take a step back and listen to your body, seeing how you respond to different foods.

We also need to remember that, while our diet is important, the foods we eat are just one aspect of our wellbeing. Health is also interlinked with our stress levels, choice of career, fitness and the relationships in our life.

The first step is to load up on superfoods for youthfulness. These are the ones to add to your shopping list:

Green, leafy vegetables, such as spinach and kale, have earned their superfood status for a good reason. The water, vitamins, minerals, and phytonutrients found in these highly nutritious foods boost blood circulation throughout the body, including the skin.

Our favourite green friends are also packed with antioxidant rich vitamins that protect against oxidative stress. Eating a diet rich in greens will not only give you beautiful, clear skin, but will also help to balance out blood sugar levels, too.

1. One of my favourite greens is Swiss chard, which is high in the antioxidant beta carotene, as well as Vitamin A, C and Vitamin K, which protect the brain and nourishes the skin. It also contains at least 13 polyphenols, while the beautiful, deep red colour of its stalks and leaves comes from a potent antioxidant. It's also full of indole-3-carbinol, which has attracted great interest for its nutrition density. Because of this, try dosing up on Swiss chard one or two times a week.

2. Bok Choy, also known as Chinese cabbage, has the appearance of a very average, pretty ordinary vegetable. Yet, when you see what lies beneath, you'll soon realise that it's an amazing, green superfood and perfect for tossing into your stir-fry or curries for an extra boost.

For starters, it has over 70 antioxidants and vitamins and minerals, including potassium, magnesium, calcium, selenium, copper, manganese, folate, choline and carotenoids. A pretty impressive haul, don't you think?

Bok Choy also contains several carotenoids, including beta carotene, lutein and zeaxanthin. While these carotenoids convert to form Vitamin A, if you have sufficient amounts of this vitamin in the body, then the carotenoids will keep circulating, mopping up free radicals along their way. Bok Choy is another of those super greens to contain indole-3-carbinol.

3. Beets are rich in folate, manganese, potassium and magnesium. Their deep and beautiful colour comes from bucketloads of the antioxidant betalain, which can clean up inflammation-causing free radicals.

Beets are also super skin savers, helping to ease dry skin and reducing pigmentation. This rocking root can even rejuvenate the complexion and can help to treat acne, too.

Better yet, you can roast them, juice them, grate them, and chuck them into desserts (think beet brownies – yum!) – beets are versatile and delicious, however you serve them!

4. Broccoli is a powerhouse of antioxidants with flavonoids, carotenoids, vitamins and minerals. Together, these work to fight off nasty free radicals to slow down skin ageing. One particular ingredient found in these leafy green trees, glucoraphanin, helps to renew skin cells and repair skin damage.

However, to maintain as many of the nutrients as possible, you should steam broccoli and, when buying, choose the deepest green florets. This is because the darkest, greenest stalks contain higher levels of carotenoids than the paler branches.

5. Berries may be tiny, but they pack a pretty hefty punch. In fact, these delicious, juicy fruits are nutritional powerhouses. All dark-skinned berries contain large amounts of antioxidants and anti-inflammatories, including quercetin. Quercetin is particularly powerful and fights inflammation throughout the whole body.

Wherever you can, try to eat fresh, organic berries. However, if cost is an issue, the freezing process does little to damage their potency, and they work out far kinder to our wallets!

Here are some of my favourite berries:
- Dried Goji berries are easy to find in larger supermarkets and health food shops. These bright red berries have been used in India for thousands of years to boost energy levels, support vision and improve sleep and kidney function.
- Blueberries have been shown to help with concentration and energy levels.
- Raspberries are high in Vitamin C, quercetin and also gallic and ellagic acid. Both of these acids help to fight cancer and are powerful anti-inflammatories.

- Strawberries boost immunity and are high in potassium, manganese and folate, which is essential for healthy DNA and cell division.

6. Celery has been shown to reduce blood pressure, and is also a fantastic antioxidant and anti-inflammatory. Recent studies show that it can even help to reduce inflammation in the digestive tract. What's more, it has mild diuretic properties, which can help to eliminate puffiness in the eyes and jaw line. Say goodbye to a tired, weary face!

   If you're not eating celery raw or juicing it and blending into smoothies, then steaming is the best method to prepare. I also recommend planting celery seeds, since the seedlings make an amazing addition to salads.

7. Pineapple is a delicious source of vitamins, copper and manganese. It has many antioxidants which work to fight off modern-day inflammatory diseases and it also contains bromelain, a special digestive enzyme which is believed to stop blood platelets building up on the walls of blood vessels. Meanwhile, our juicy, tropical friend is also rich in Vitamin C to reduce inflammatory skin conditions. Now, where's that pina colada...?

8. Salmon is renowned for being a fantastic source of Omega-3, which is thought to reduce inflammation in our joints and prevent heart disease. These same Omega-3s make it an excellent skin food, and it's also rich in DMAE (dimethylaminoethanol) to naturally firm the skin.

   As well as this, salmon contains special bioactive peptides which are beneficial for our bones and joints. By enjoying fish or seafood once a week, we can even lower our risk of cognitive decline as we age.

9. Mushrooms may be cheap, but they are most definitely not ordinary! Marvelous mushrooms are an excellent source of selenium, copper, niacin, potassium and phosphorous. However, their cell walls are indigestible until heated, so make sure you cook your mushrooms first to really reap the rewards.

   Another clever thing about these funny little fungi is that they can mop up excess oestrogen in the body, which make them potential warriors in the fight against breast cancer. In fact, an early stage tissue culture study published in November 2010 in the 'Experimental Biology and Medicine Journal' found that white button mushrooms, along with four other varieties, significantly suppressed breast cancer cell growth and reproduction.

   Of course, there needs to be more work carried out in this area before we can really sing their praises. Yet, mushrooms are also rich in beta-glucans, which gives our immune system some muscles to fight off colds, flu and viruses, and they also contain a polysaccharide that can hydrate and plump the skin.

10. Nuts are one of your complexion's best friends! They are packed full of body-loving fats which are amazing for keeping our skin super nourished.

     In fact, reaching for a small handful of nuts at snack time can also do incredible things for your body by improving blood sugar and cholesterol levels. And, really, you can take your pick of nuts – they all have benefits, and are rich in Vitamin E and magnesium. They're also a fantastic source of protein for vegetarians and vegans. And, as an extra top tip, if you find nuts difficult to digest, try soaking them in water overnight.

     While all nuts are good for us, my favourites include walnuts, almonds and Brazil nuts. Funny, wrinkly little walnuts are rich in Omega-3 for brain, heart and skin health – they even look like miniature brains!

     Meanwhile, almonds are high in Vitamin E, arginine, magnesium, copper, manganese, calcium and potassium, which are all key nutrients for heart health. They also support healthy cholesterol and blood pressure levels. Being Vitamin E rich, too, makes them an excellent food for skin.

     Finally, Brazil nuts aren't just to be saved for dark chocolate! They give us the richest source of selenium, which is hard to find in other foods. Selenium helps to balance out our mood (meaning Brazil nuts are ideal for certain times of the month), and is an excellent anti-inflammatory. Research has also shown that there is a link between a thyroid metabolism and selenium deficiency.

11. Turmeric is wonderful for adding earthiness, colour and vibrancy to your dishes. Yet this super spice is also an incredibly powerful anti-inflammatory and comes with heaps of health benefits.

     In fact, turmeric has been used for centuries as a natural remedy since it has many healing properties, which are often credited to its high levels of curcumin. However, studies have shown that even without curcumin, turmeric can work its healing magic.

     You see, turmeric is also high in natural fatty acids, which slow down the speed the liver processes them at by 7-8 percent (curcumin is lacking in these fats). What's more, curcumin forms just 5 percent of the turmeric root, and there are over 300 other important ingredients in the remaining 95 percent. While these other components haven't received the same microscopic attention that curcumin has, some may be just as good for us – if not better!

Studies have shown that, as well as being antibacterial, a generous sprinkling of turmeric can help with:
- The immune system
- Healthy blood sugar levels
- Liver function
- Cognitive function

- Skin health, including reducing acne
- Inflammation
- Brain health
- Joint health
- A healthy lymphatic system
- Keeping our digestive system healthy
- Gall bladder function
- Overall wellbeing

Yet, before you stockpile on the homemade curries, turmeric is fairly versatile, and there are heaps of ways to use this beautiful spice!

Used in curries, it is wonderfully warming in hot drinks and even homemade, healthier cookies. Another useful tip is to use it alongside a sprinkling of black pepper, which can slow the liver's metabolisation of turmeric, meaning it stays in the blood stream longer.

Amazingly, black pepper can even increase the availability of turmeric by up to 2,000 percent. Yes, 2,000!

My favourite way to enjoy turmeric is by mixing a teaspoon of powdered turmeric to four teaspoons of yoghurt, alongside a sprinkle of black pepper. It doesn't sound nice, but it is more palatable than you might think, and packs enormous health benefits. If possible, try using raw, grated turmeric root – but remember to wear rubber gloves first to avoid bright yellow hands!

12. Spicy, delicious ginger is part of the same plant family as turmeric, and can work small miracles on our digestive system.

The amazing thing is that there are 115 different chemical components hiding in the ginger root, and we can get some pretty impressive benefits from its antioxidants called gingerols. These aptly-named antioxidants help to prevent blood clots, and can protect us from both heart attacks and strokes.

Want to reap the rewards? You can easily get a ginger fix – and, no, you don't need to reach for a gingernut biscuit! The best way to enjoy this spice is by drinking ginger tea, or by grating fresh ginger root into a stir fry or smoothie.

13. We should all be sprinkling versatile super seeds, including chia, sunflower, pumpkin and flax seeds, into our diet. These tiny little wonders are all rich in Omega-3s and phytonutrients, so they're important for both super skin and even our well-being.

Sunflower seeds are delicious mixed into homemade granola or sprinkled over our morning bowl of porridge, and are high in vitamins B & E, copper, phosphorous and selenium. They also hide pretty hefty amounts of vitamin E, which helps to reduce the risk of heart disease.

Similarly, pumpkin seeds are rich in protein and Vitamin E. Clever chia seeds are rich in zinc, potassium, fibre and omega fatty acids. They're also a wonderful source of plant-based protein, which makes them a great addition to vegan or vegetarian diets. Plus, if you've never made a chia pudding before, you're in for a real treat!

Finally, flax have all the benefits of other seeds, but are also incredibly high in lignans, which helps to promote healthy cholesterol levels.

14. Garlic may well be our favourite herb at Rejuvenated HQ. In fact, we seem to add it to just about every meal, yet we often forget about the incredible health benefits that it contains! However, garlic comes a pretty close second to turmeric in terms of body-loving, health-boosting properties.

Allicin is just one of garlic's marvellous medicinal components, and is anti-inflammatory and antibacterial. It can even increase the body's level of antioxidants!

The large amount of allicin found in garlic also means that it is anti-fungal and full of anti-ageing, smoothing goodness for the skin. Other studies have revealed it can protect us against heart disease, cancer, strokes and infections.

15. Delicious kombucha and fermented foods, including kimchi, kefir and sauerkraut, can all increase the happy, friendly bacteria in our gut. In turn, this can help to keep our digestive system happy, support weight loss and supercharge the immune system.

Here in the Western world, we are only just starting to understand the benefits of fermented foods in our diet, so if you don't know where to start, my favourites include:

- Kombucha, which is a tasty drink made from black or green tea. However, you can grow your own from a starter 'scoby', or simply buy a bottle from a health food store.
- Kefir is fermented from milk to produce a yoghurt-type drink.
- Kimchi, a pickled cabbage dish from Korea, tastes delicious with stir-fries or Asian-inspired cuisine.
- A spoonful of sauerkraut, a pickled cabbage dish from Germany and Austria, is full of body boosters, and is cheap and simple to make, too!

Why are fermented foods important?

So, why are these fermented foods so good for us? And why should we be eating them? Well, to keep things short and sweet, the key to their importance lies in our gut.

Over the last decade, science has honed in on the importance of our tums and digestive system when it comes to the fight against inflammation. This fledgling work has revealed that inflammatory diseases, as well as the health of our brain, our moods and even our weight, could all be influenced by the balance of good and bad bacteria within our gut.

Thanks to this work, a medical revolution is under way to help us to understand these little microbes and the microbiome that they live in.

However, one thing we do know is this: the huge numbers of organisms lurking within our gut outnumbers our cells by ten to one, with over 400 known species. Bacteria, meanwhile, isn't all bad – we can get the good, the bad and the downright ugly.

As you now know, our so-called 'good' bacteria have all sorts of benefits for our body. Yet the problem is, our beneficial bacteria can come and go, and modern day life can throw our tummies out of synch further still. In fact, each of these can wreak havoc on our gut flora:

- Antibiotics
- Diets low in fermentable fibres
- Chronic stress
- Chronic infections
- Diets high in refined foods

Because of this, it's important that we take steps to support our inner gut, and we can give them a head start with our diets.

To restore and rebalance your gut flora, you should:

- Eat fermented foods, like those we talked about above
- Enjoy fermentable fibres, including sweet potato, yucca and yams
- Remove toxins from the diet
- Reduce stress

Can a low fodmap diet help IBS?

From bloating and gas to stomach aches and pains, IBS is a problem that affects all too many of us. Yet, if you're one of the many people who suffer from this sometime debilitating condition, there are answers – it's all about finding what works for you.

More and more, people are discovering that a low-FODMAP diet can help those with digestive woes. While it might sound complicated, let me put it into English for you. Or, at least, I'll try!

Put simply, FODMAPS (Fermentable, Oligo-, Di, Monosaccharides and Polyols, to be a little more technical) are short chain carbohydrates some of us find hard to digest. FODMAPs are naturally present in certain foods, including some we see as 'healthy', yet for some of us, they may trigger nasty irritable bowel symptoms.

These foods can include lactose, which is found in dairy, fructose and other sweet foods, sorbitol and some vegetables such as onions, garlics and leeks.

If you are interested in reading more, then there are lots of apps which are full of advice and support, as well as handy shopping lists of high and low-FODMAP foods. If you're in doubt, then try avoiding foods with high FODMAP scores for a week to see if they're causing an imbalance.

How to deconstruct your food cravings

For many of us – especially the food-loving ones, like me! – the hardest thing when you start any new eating programme is dealing with food cravings. Whether you love your sweets or chocolate, or you have a taste for salty crisps and nuts, there are always foods that we reach for when we are low, or feeling under the weather.

The problem is, most of our comfort foods are ones which cause inflammation, and they're also the ones we crave and miss when we're embarking on a new healthy eating regime.

So, why is this? Well, the brain releases a chemical called dopamine, which is a clever little neurotransmitter that triggers the brain's reward and pleasure centres. Many people get addicted to something because it gives them instant gratification, a surge in happiness, and these addictions could be caused by low levels of dopamine.

Yet, it doesn't always have to be this way! Instead, there are plenty of other things you can do to help boost levels. Here are some of my top tips:

Do something different

If you're a creature of habit and find yourself reaching for a glass of wine or the biscuit tin come 8pm, then try mixing up your routine. You could book a yoga class or go for a walk, both of which will release happy-boosting endorphins.

If that doesn't tickle your fancy, then get creative! You could even try listening to music, which can increase dopamine levels and motivate you to exercise. I promise that it can work wonders!

If you do find yourself struggling, then try not to feel disheartened. The worst of the cravings will be over within three days, so be super kind to yourself in the first 96 hours – it will get better.

And, in the meantime, here's how you can beat those cravings and turn on the longevity factor:

If You're Craving...Fatty Foods

Whether you have a hankering for fried chicken or cheese, there is a cure for fatty food cravings. In fact, a craving of these foods could simply be a sign that your body is deficient in Omega-3 essential fatty acids, which help to transport substances in and out of our cells.

If you often find yourself lusting after fatty foods, then try taking an Omega-3 supplement to help to reduce cravings for fatty foods. Our Rejuvenated Aliol is perfect for this since it is sourced from algae and suitable for all diets.

If You're Craving...Chocolate

I think most of us are guilty of this at some point, and it's probably the biggest addiction in the Western world. After all, how many of us will reach for a bar of chocolate (or two!) after a bad day at work?

Of course, one of the reasons for this is simply down to the sweet, addictive sugar content. However, it could also be that your body is lacking in magnesium. Magnesium is one of the busiest minerals in our body as it activates over 300 chemical reactions, yet a lack of it can leave us feeling tired and lethargic.

To kick that chocolate habit and to give magnesium levels a boost, try snacking on nuts and eating more pulses, which are both rich in this mineral. Our very own H3O Hydration and H30 Night Repair is also rich in magnesium, so these are handy weapons to have to hand, too.

And, for when nothing but chocolate will do, aim to have a stash of good quality dark chocolate hidden away, ideally with 75% or more cacao solids. A couple of squares will soon see that urge satisfied.

If You're Craving...Sugar

Let's face it, we all know that we should be eating less sugar, that it's public enemy number one when it comes to our diets. Yet, it's not always that easy – for most people it still makes up a third of our diet.

This is partly because the white stuff is super addictive and can cause huge rollercoasters in our blood sugar levels. These troughs and peaks lead us to crave more and more sweet stuff, and can ultimately lead to Type II diabetes and adrenal problems.

If you're worried about your sugar intake, then try adding good quality protein to all of your meals. For example, you could try starting the day by breakfasting on eggs or fish instead of high-carb, sugar-laden cereals, and eating more sweet veggies, such as carrots and sweet potatoes.

Instead of snacking on biscuits or wandering to the vending machine, you could also try a small handful of nuts, or a few cubes of creamy goat's cheese. The dark chocolate trick I mentioned above works a treat, too!

Since we often crave sweet things and become irritable when we're pre-menstrual, it may also help to take a Vitamin B6 supplement (200 mg per day) to boost our 'feel good' hormone prostaglandin E1.

If You're Craving...Salt

When you find yourself unable to resist a family bag of crisps at the petrol station, is it really the taste that you can't resist, or is it simply your body trying to deal with stressful situations? You see, salt blunts our body's natural response to stress by lowering the production of stress hormones.

Instead of eating salty chips or crisps, though, there are other ways to curb those cravings. You could try dealing with stressful situations by enjoying yoga or meditation – and, if you still want salt on your food, try a sprinkling of Himalayan pink salt crystals, which contain a healthy balance of minerals.

If You're Craving...Carbs

From buttery toast to huge bowlfuls of pasta, carbs are one of the best comfort foods around. The reason why is fairly simple – carbohydrates stimulate the happy hormone, serotonin.

Of course, this why we often reach for those foods that remind us of our childhood when we're feeling low, such as potatoes, white bread and pasta. Yet it could also mean that our lust for carbs comes from low levels of serotonin and endorphins.

If you're feeling the need for carbs (and, by this, I don't mean delicious, nutritious complex carbs!), try to eat protein first, which will help to balance insulin production and stop you from over-eating carbohydrates. Next, ditch those processed carbs and reach for our favourite slow-release carbohydrates, instead. Foods such as sweet potatoes, oats and pulses will keep you fuller for longer.

Another handy way to kill carb cravings is to get sweaty! Exercise boosts serotonin and endorphin levels, so pull on your trainers, get outside and take a long walk.

If You're Craving...Caffeine

How many of you use coffee or caffeine as a prop? As something to simply see you through those long meetings at work, or to wake you up in the morning?

Many of us are guilty of this! We treat coffee as rocket fuel, drinking it to keep us stimulated and alert. However, the truth is it often leaves us more exhausted than ever before.

If you're drinking too much caffeine, then there are alternatives. Instead of automatically putting on the kettle, take a break, have five minutes of calm and even put your head down. An early night can also work wonders, and you don't need me to remind you of the boost it can give your skin, too!

If you still can't do without your caffeine fix, then consider alternatives such as green tea. I love sipping on a hot matcha tea, which is full of antioxidants and is known to boost the metabolism, too.

WEEK 2

LET'S HYDRATE!

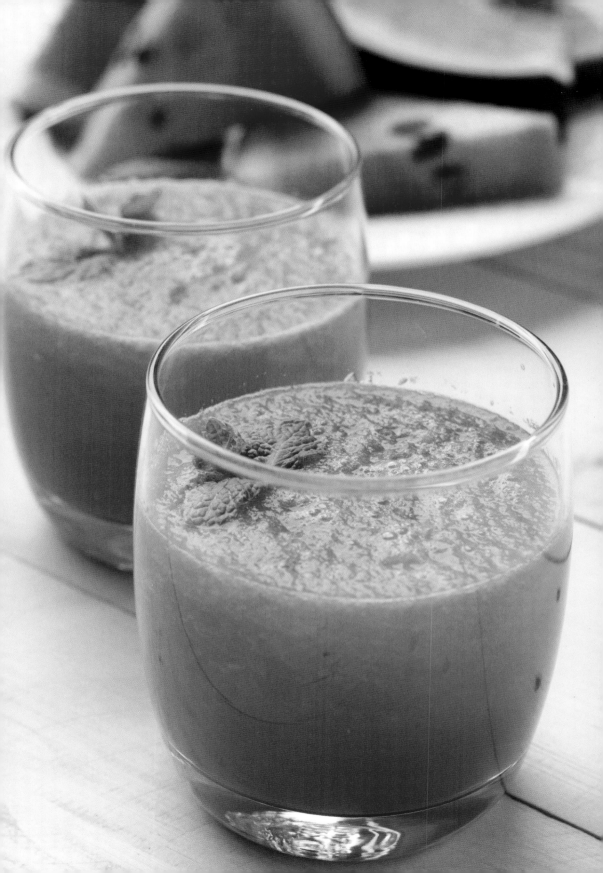

'You are not just what you eat, you are what you drink.'

– Dr Batnabgelidj

Now that we're into your second week of Rejuvenated, it's time to ramp that water intake right up and stay hydrated!

While it may not seem all that important, simple, wonderful water is the very cornerstone of our lives – we simply can't live without it. Water is our body's most important nutrient, and is actually 50-70 per cent of our body weight.

Because of this, low-levels of fluid can cause inflammation in our bodies, while chronic, long-term dehydration can trigger all sorts of diseases. Yet, in spite of this, many of us don't drink anywhere enough of this precious nutrient, even though it's so freely available – all we have to do is turn on the tap!

Now that you've made some changes to your lifestyle, I'd like you to focus on one more: getting into healthy drinking habits. You could start your day by drinking water as soon as you get up, or perhaps you could sip on a hot water with a squeeze of lemon. Whatever you do, aim to drink some more!

If you're a caffeine addict, then don't worry – there's an easy solution for you, too! If you normally boil the kettle for endless cups of tea and coffee, aim to substitute every alternate one with a glass of water, or try switching to herbal and fruit teas, instead. Both your body and skin will soon be reaping the rewards!

Why do i need water?

Precious H20 is vital for our health. Although we can go for several weeks without food, our bodies lose large amounts of water every day, making it impossible to survive without it.

Staying hydrated keeps all of our organs ticking along happily, and supports our body's digestive, circulatory and excretory functions. We also need it to keep all those water-absorbable vitamins and nutrients whizzing through our blood stream and cells.

As well as this, water carries oxygen to every single cell in our bodies. It transports sodium, calcium, magnesium, potassium and other salts to our cells for electrolyte balance, which we need to function properly and healthily.

When we're drinking plenty, the blood and lymphatic fluid can flow more easily. Blood carries enzymes and nutrients to the organs, while the lymph fluid can help to flush away waste and toxins.

Yet, I'm still not finished! Wonderful water also helps to dilute acids in the body, making the blood more alkaline and our insides stronger and healthier. It can moisturise and plump up our skin, making it look younger and fresher, and it's also essential for brain health.

We sometimes forget that the brain is an organ too – one that's almost entirely made up of water and fat. Water fluid cushions every joint and bone in the body, and every single vertebrae is also surrounded by it. This means that if you want a healthy, pain-free back, you need to get drinking!

So, you can see water is a pretty magical ingredient. The most magical, precious one accessible to us, in fact. Even more important than those so-called superfoods, such as kale and beetroot. Yet, if all of that was a lot to take in, then simply scan this instead to see why H2O is so important:

Why we need water:

- Helps kidneys to excrete acids
- Relieves stress
- Reduces bad cholesterol levels
- Stabilises blood pressure
- Prevents headaches
- Helps to prevent hangovers
- Eases fatigue
- Helps to halt allergic reactions
- Prevents dehydration and dryness of the skin

Just in case you're not sure if you need to drink more, then here are some of the classic symptoms of dehydration:

- Dark yellow urine (pale urine is healthy)
- Constipation
- Skin flare-ups
- Hunger
- Mood swings
- Fatigue
- Lots of joint problems

What is cellular water?

Are you ready to discover more about our precious H2O? Pour yourself a glass of ice cold water, add a squeeze of lemon, and read on...

Of the total water in our bodies, two thirds is intracellular water, which is the H20 content found within our cells. Meanwhile, extracellular water is body water found outside our cells, and it's an increase in this which can cause excess weight and swelling or bloating in the limbs.

The problem is, fluctuations in our hormones, as well as with our protein and mineral levels, can all cause an imbalance and lead to high blood pressure.

Can I improve the balance of my cellular water?

Happily, yes! Here at Rejuvenated, we have an easy-to-follow strategy to help with this.

First of all, we need to strengthen the cell walls. Once we've done this, it's important that we work on supporting the ways in which we get water across the cell membrane for healthy fluid balance.

Our collagen drink, Collagen Shots, can help by providing all the amino acids we need to contribute to building healthy cell walls, while our H30 Hydration can help to balance fluid levels, too.

H3O Hydration is a special hypotonic drink which allows for speedy transmission of electrolytes and minerals through the stomach wall, into the blood stream and on to the cells.

How much water should I drink?

Well, quite a lot! And probably more than you're drinking right now.

While there's never been a clinical study to show that you actually need to drink two litres of water a day, most scientists and dieticians agree that we should be sipping plenty of fluids throughout the day.

Just how much we need depends on each person, and how active we are, too. It will also fluctuate according to the time of year – our bodies need much less in the winter than during a sizzling hot summer heatwave.

Of course, while water is your healthiest, most refreshing option, tea and coffee, although slightly dehydrating, also contributes to our daily intake.

Eat your water

If you don't find it easy to drink up, then try eating up instead to hydrate your body. Foods like cucumber, melon and strawberries are incredibly high in water.

Does dehydration affect your skin?

We always hear skin specialists and celebrities preaching that we need to drink up for healthy, glowing skin. While there are all sorts of lotions and potions to combat dehydration, water is the cheapest – and most effective – tool we have.

Just take a moment to think: if your skin is dehydrated on the outside, then what's it like on the inside? True cellular hydration starts from within?

If you feel like your skin needs a helping hand to get that glow, then read on:

How can cellular hydration help the skin?

If life were simple, we'd be able to just slather on a cream to correct our dehydrated skin. Of course, life isn't simple, and that's not the complete answer.

While moisturising is important, drinking enough fluids is crucial in keeping our skin looking fresh and youthful (although, again, it's not the complete answer). Of course, there can also be too much of a good thing – high volumes of water can cause bloating and frequent trips to the loo!

Yet, when you consider that our skin is the last organ to benefit from water intake, you'll soon see why it's tricky to achieve super-charged, plump skin through water alone.

This is where the Natural Moisture Factor comes in to play...

What does the Natural Moisture Factor do?

Have you ever noticed how some people just glow – the secret is the Natural Moisture Factor. This is how you can get the fresh and radiant skin you've always dreamed of.

Our superficial, outer layer of the skin – the Stratum Corneum – contains a unique collection of 'naturally-occurring humectants'. Together, these are known as the Natural Moisturising Factor (NMF) and have the special super power to attract and bind with water.

The Natural Moisture Factor does an incredible job of regulating skin hydration, and can do all sorts of clever things:

- Reduce the forces that bind and harden keratin fibres to boost and maintain skin elasticity.
- Allow enzymes to break down dead skin cells to reveal fresher, healthier skin.
- Protect the natural barrier function of skin.

For a long time, we believed that this outer skin layer was biologically dead. Essentially it is, but it still has a unique dynamic structure where enzymes are active and need water to thrive.

If we have a healthy Natural Moisture Factor, we can simply provide this water by attracting it from the atmosphere via its abundance of amino acids and minerals. In fact, its absorption of water is so efficient, so good, that NMF virtually dissolves itself within the water drawn to the surface.

Another handy thing about NMF is that it supports a healthy water balance in our outer skin layer, which stops an excess of water from entering the skin.

WEEK 3

Strength & Flexibility

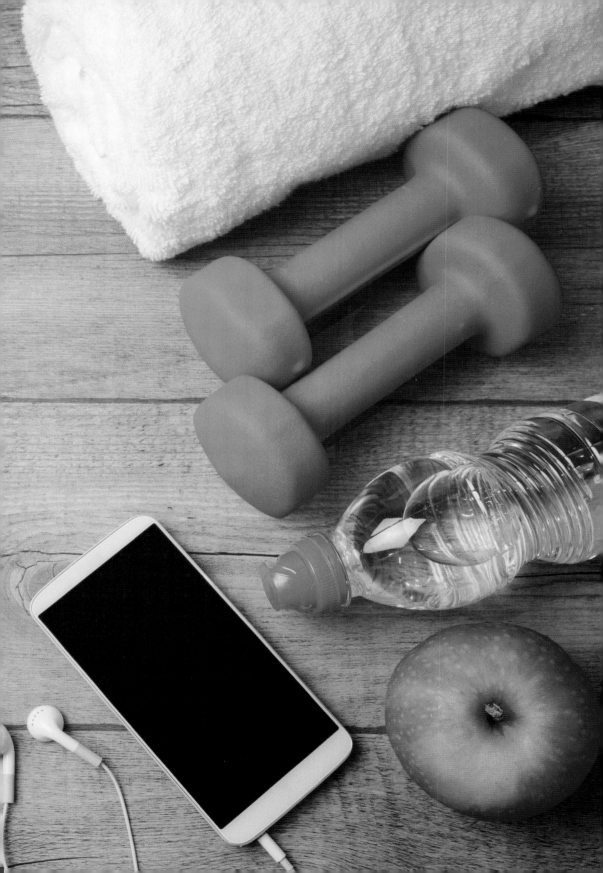

Strength & Flexibility

Whether you want to dance, run, walk, swim or climb mountains, staying active is just as important for our bodies as eating healthily.

I know that sometimes it can be hard to exercise, but we've all been designed to move, and endless studies have shown that our bodies go downhill pretty quickly when we're inactive for long stretches.

Of course, in between juggling relationships, children, hectic social lives or busy workdays, it can be difficult to squeeze in the time to work out. Yet, you don't need to pound a treadmill for hours at the gym to see results! Studies show that just 150 minutes – that's two and a half hours – of moderate exercise a week can raise our life expectancy by five years.

That's little over 20 minutes a day, and can be something as simple and as easy as pulling on your trainers and heading out for a powerwalk! Fairly tempting, isn't it it? Especially when you consider the alternative.

Plus, when you throw in the fact that sitting for six or more hours a day can have a negative effect on the body (and, let's face it, working in an office can easily see us do this), it's more important than ever before to get moving to reduce the impact.

I understand that not everyone likes to exercise, though! If you're not that much into working out, the secret is do something that you enjoy and that fits in to your lifestyle – it doesn't usually work if you decide that you're going to go from couch potato to running five miles a day!

You don't have to run a marathon to be fitter and healthier, and it doesn't matter if you're not sporty. The key is to move your body and to try different things until you find what works for you.

Another secret is to choose the best time of day to work out. I'm very much a morning person, so I like to get my routine done first thing, and then I can forget about it for the rest of the day, or top up later if I want to. You might be an afternoon or evening person, just do what works for you.

And if you're wondering what kind of exercise is good for you, then you have my permission to run free and go wild! Strength, flexibility and aerobic health are all important. Here's why:

Why should I use strength building exercises?

Long gone are the days when we thought that lifting weights would make a woman look manly and bulky. Now, it's now very much in style for a woman to have a lean, firm physique, which you can achieve by lifting weights.

Whether you're a man or woman, once you've gone through puberty, you start to lose around one percent of bone and muscle strength each year. It sounds pretty scary, but don't be too concerned – you can reverse it by adding strength training to your exercise programme.

What's more, lifting weights can boost energy levels and raise those endorphins to give you a feel-good factor. And you don't need to reach for those huge weights in the gym to see the benefits, too – you can use light dumbbells, bottles of water or even your own body weight to get started.

Here's why else you should start lifting:

- Lose weight
- Strengthen bones
- Improve heart health
- Improve balance and posture

Sounds pretty impressive, doesn't it? I also love how strong and empowered I feel when I've lifted weights. Let's get lifting!

Flexibility and posture:

Our flexibility and posture usually deteriorate with age, but this doesn't have to be the case for you! It is possible to boost your flexibility and be like a gymnast, even well into your so-called later years.

Stretches with exercises such as yoga and Pilates can help to strengthen the body, make your limbs longer and leaner, and boost flexibility. Happily, flexibility is important for mobility and can reduce those niggling aches and pains, too.

Want to give it a go? Try incorporating stretching into your work-out to maintain mobility and reduce the potential for injury. If you suffer from tension, focus on your shoulders and neck but also include hips, thighs, calves and lower back. If you're unsure about what to do, you could try taking a yoga class at least once a week, although two to three classes are ideal.

Another one of my tips for super long, flexible limbs is to limit the time that you wear high heels, particularly if you spend most of the day on your feet. They might make you feel good, but high heels change the way your body is aligned and affect your back and posture.

The scientific reasons to do aerobic exercise

Getting sweaty and jumping around is proven to strengthen our heart and our lungs. As well as this, it can help to lower cholesterol and blood sugar levels and boost the immune system. It can even send our metabolism soaring for up to 24 hours after working out, meaning you burn off more calories, and can squeeze into those skinny jeans even quicker!

The thing is, when you move your limbs faster than your body is used to, you start to breathe faster and more deeply. This increases the amount of oxygen in the blood, and so your heart has to beat faster and work harder to pump that blood back to your muscles. As well as this, those happy-boosting endorphins also get released to make you feel good, and to reduce stress.

What is fascia and how does it impact your health?

I hope that's convinced you to dust off those trainers and treat yourself to some exercise gear. Yet, if you're still frowning at your book and feeling a little bit cynical, then let me introduce you to fascia, and how it can affect your health.

Do you ever wake up feeling stiff, finding that you simply can't get your body moving? Or try to stand up after an evening snuggled on the sofa, only to discover that your back is aching and refusing to move with ease? If you answered 'yes', then it might be that your body fascia needs smoothing out.

Our fascia is the biological fabric that keeps us together. It's a network of connective tissues that are made up of tightly packed-in protein fibres. This sheet of tissue weaves throughout the entire body, connecting and supporting every muscle, bone and even our organs.

These fascias work with our muscles, too, helping entire muscle groups to communicate with one another. A healthy fascia allows us to move with grace and ease (think ballerina-esque movement) and can also help to maximise our exercise performance.

In an ideal world, each of us will have a fascia that is soft and supple so that it can glide and twist like long, thin sheets of rubber. Yet, when it becomes dehydrated or damaged, the strands don't function correctly and can lead to inflammation and pain.

Long periods of inactivity can also cause our fascia to become rigid and stiff. If you do feel a bit Zombie-like after a good night's sleep, the best way to loosen it up is to stretch out those arms and legs, before rolling gently from side to side. Once you've done that, ease yourself out of bed nice and slowly to gently coax the strands apart.

To keep your fascia supple throughout the day, you could try gently massaging any sore points and stiff areas with a foam roller or yoga ball, or simple stretch and walk around. This is a real treat for the body, and prevents aches and strains from building up. A good massage therapist can also help to relieve tension – the gentle Bowen technique is particularly beneficial, and can smooth and release our fascia.

Finally, you can free up that fascia and keep it performing well by boosting collagen and hydration levels. You can do this by adding the Rejuvenated products to your daily routine.

Are you ready?

I hope I've convinced you that exercise can truly transform both your body and your mind!

Don't worry, though, you don't need to run marathons to get started. I'm no athlete but, for my body and I, it works to combine yoga with walking and light weights. An ideal week could include a swim or a few brisk walks. If you're a team player, then try playing a game with a group of people – you'll love the friendship and bonds you form!

Alternatively, you could take two or three classes of yoga and do a couple of sessions of light weights. There's no need for expensive club fees to keep fit, but if you find it motivates you to get out of the door, then go for it! The £30 monthly fee will prove to be more than worth it.

Get started:

Start with small, baby steps rather than giant leaps and unrealistic goals, and make sure you check with your doctor first if you've been inactive for a while, or are carrying an injury. You could start with short walks and build up from there.

I also find it helps to set myself goals, imagining how I'll feel in 30 days' time if I start out now and stick with things. You could try picturing yourself slipping into that dress you've been admiring for a while, or thinking of yourself stronger, firmer and leaner, and with bags more energy.

If you find this hard, try pinning yourself little notes and motivational messages around the house to help you to get there. Trust me, this makes exercising much, much easier on those days when you're really not feeling it!

And, if you're still doubting yourself, then don't: I know you can do it. All it takes is focus and two and a half to four hours a week, and I guarantee that you'll feel the best, most vibrant version of you.

Small steps with big rewards:

Another of my get fit tips is to invest in a pedometer (don't worry, they don't have to break the bank – you can buy them for under £20) or a smart watch to monitor how much activity you're doing throughout the day, without even stepping into the gym. You might surprise yourself with just how far you actually walk!

If you're falling a little short of your daily step target (I try to aim for 10,000 steps each day), then try hopping off the bus a stop earlier than normal, or parking your car a little further away from your destination and finishing your journey on foot.

Wherever you can, take the stairs instead of the lift, and enjoy mini breaks at work to get up and wander around. If you have a hands-free phone, walk around while taking calls.

And, if you're really feeling up for the challenge, then here are a few of my other tips to get moving and to become the healthiest, fittest you:

- If you love working out to music, try putting on a track that's a little more upbeat to increase your pace.
- Pop on an exercise or fitness DVD, or browse some of the free fitness channels on YouTube. For low intensity workouts, try Rodney Yee Yoga or the Tracey Anderson Mat Workout (Tracey is the coach that body-conscious celebs turn to, so you know you'll be in good hands!). If you like the current HIIT trend (high-intensity interval training), then give Joe Wicks or Jillian Michaels a try, but be mindful that these can be quite intense.

However, whatever it is that you want to try, just a quick note of caution from us first: always check with your doctor or medical practitioner before you dive head-first into a new fitness programme.

Now, go dust off those trainers, and get moving!

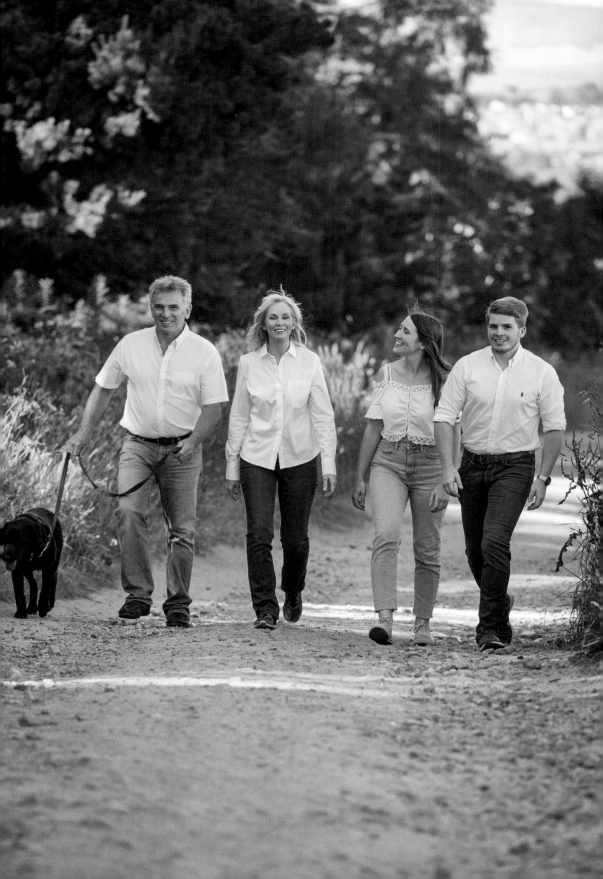

WEEK 4

Sleep & Relaxation

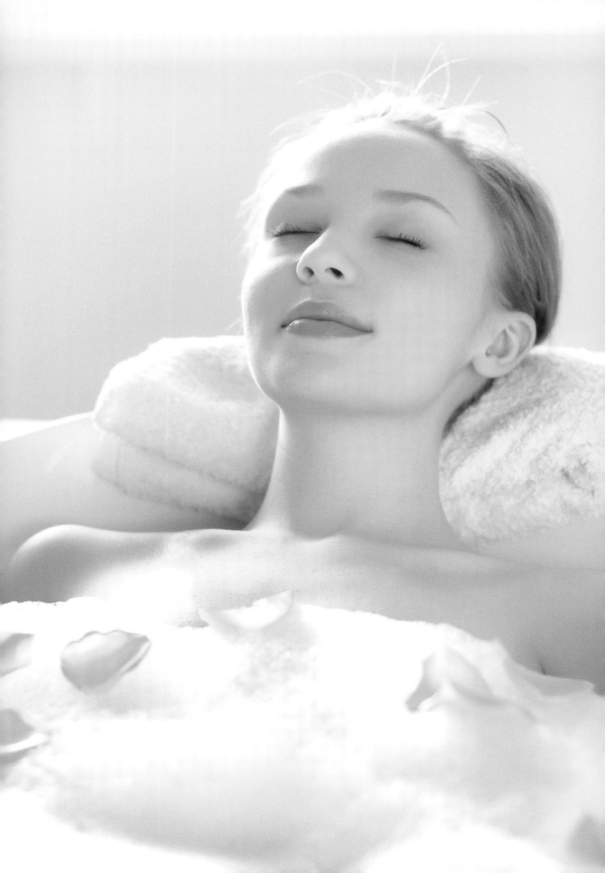

The Secret To Sleep And Relaxation

We all know that getting plenty of sleep can boost our body, mind and glow. Yet, when you're manic at work or feeling fretful, it's not always that simple.

So, just how do you ease into good sleeping habits and ensure you're feeling rested, recharged and revitalised? Well, I'd like you to meet the YOGA CIRCADIAN RYTHM - MYSTERY, the secret to fantastic sleep and relaxation...

Do you find yourself nodding off while you're watching the TV, but then lying awake for hours when you do finally clamber into bed? Tossing and turning, you're still awake three hours later and in desperate need of a trip to the loo. And that's then followed by another hour of tossing and turning!

If this sounds like you, then, come the morning, chances are that you're exhausted, grumpy and sluggish when the alarm goes off. In fact, you may well feel even more tired than you did before you went to bed, and I'll bet that you often hit snooze on the clock, too!

The thing is, we need to prioritise sleep every bit as much as we do exercise and healthy eating. You see, good quality sleep lets our body recharge and heal, and it also has an anti-inflammatory effect – this is why bad sleep patterns leave us more susceptible to infection and can lead to inflammation.

Yet, is a good night's sleep really such a mystery?
Well, unfortunately, for many of us, yes it is.

In the 21st century, we've made some truly amazing scientific discoveries and built some incredible structures, but our bodies work pretty much the same as they always have, and beat to a primal clock.

We're all controlled by circadian rhythms, which govern each of our physical, mental and behavioural changes during a 24-hour day. These rhythms respond to light and darkness, or day and night. Yet, they can be fooled – something as simple as the LED digital time on a clock, or the light from our phones, can trigger the rhythm, telling us it's time to get up.

What many people don't realise is that our sleep patterns follow a series of 90-minute cycles, and we all need around four to five of these sleep cycles a night. Of course, we are all different, but seven and a half hours or five cycles of sleep is a good rule of thumb.

However, with today's lifestyle, that can seem like Mission: Impossible. This is where putting a sleep plan in place may help you, and could even transform your life.

Sleep and metabolism

Did you know that sleep actually plays a big part in a healthy, happy metabolism?

Some of us may know this all too well. You seem to be doing everything right, eating healthily and hitting the gym, yet those pounds still keep on creeping up. If that sounds all too familiar, then it could be that your sleep situation needs examining first.

To lose out on sleep for the odd night is OK, but if you miss out on shut eye too often, then it can do damage to more than just your weight balance. Here are the facts on how those late nights affect your overall wellbeing:

- A recent study showed that getting just 30 minutes too little sleep each night can increase your risk of obesity and diabetes. Sleep is vital for repair and restoration to rejuvenate our body for the next day (which is why we all know the term 'beauty sleep'!) When we don't get enough, our cognitive function is impaired and our decision making, reaction time and memory all start to suffer.

- Have you ever noticed that, when you're tired, you become hungry and crave carbs? This is because exhaustion can cause the body to release a hormone called ghrelin, AKA the hunger hormone, and also reduces leptin, which tells our body when we're full.
  One study even showed that sleep-deprived participants ate on average 300 more calories per day. While that may not seem all that much, another study showed that, over the course of a week, people who slept for four or five hours rather than ten gained an extra 2lbs in weight over seven days.

- Another side effect of burning the candle at both ends is stress. With less sleep, the body goes into stress mode and releases cortisol, which also increases the appetite. As well as this, the body triggers the need for serotonin to reduce the tension. The problem is, the easiest way to raise serotonin levels is from high-fat and carb-loaded foods, so it's easy to see why you might want to raid the biscuit tin.

- As if that weren't enough to send you running for the covers, sleep deprivation can also slow down our cells' ability to process sugar, which causes a surge in body sugar levels. Long-term effects of this can lead to diabetes and heart disease.

How to set up your own sleep plan:

How do you enjoy the best sleep of your life? Ideally, your sleep plan will be consistent, but try to allow for flexibility – staying out with friends for an hour or so past bedtime for a birthday or celebration is never going to hurt!

Here are some of my ideas for a simple sleep plan, but you can be flexible and tailor them to suit you and your own needs:

1. If you need to be up early each day, work backwards to see what time you should be settling down between the sheets. For example, a 6am start should see you in bed by 10.30pm.

2. Drink plenty of fluids through the day to stay hydrated, since dehydration can cause you to wake in the middle of the night, gasping for a glass of water.

3. Cleanse, tone and moisturise your face a couple of hours before bedtime so that you're not too tired to remove make up. This will also help to give your skin time to breathe, make up free.

4. An hour or so before bedtime, take a warm bath, or do some yoga to help to lull you into a deeper, more restful sleep.

5. Don't drink alcohol or eat during the hour before you go to bed, which can keep you tossing and turning throughout the early hours.

6. Once your head has hit the pillow, let yourself have some downtime. I like to meditate or read for a short time to leave the stress of the day behind. Allow your mind some time to calm down and, if something pops into your head, then make a note and forget about it until tomorrow.

7. Kick the blue light habit! Mobile devices and tablets have given us great freedom and flexibility in both our work and personal lives. Yet, the downside is that most of us are carrying a pretty serious mobile addiction – the average person checks their device 85 times a day, while a third of us check it in the middle of the night!
   A mobile addiction is never going to be a good thing, but it can wreak havoc on our sleep, too. For starters, it's well documented that light from electronic devices can disturb sleep patterns. Try putting your phone down by 8pm every night and, if you wear a fitness device 24 hours a day, try leaving it outside the bedroom for a few nights to see if your sleep pattern improves.

8. Unless you live in a remote village or in the middle of the countryside, chances are there will be some flooding of night-time light in the bedroom. Yet, as you now know, this can stimulate those old circadian rhythms, and trick you into waking up too early. Of course, you can hardly turn out the street lights, so try buying an eye mask or investing in black-out curtains or blinds, instead.

9. If you have a dimmer switch, then turn down the lights before bedtime, since darkness naturally stimulates production of melatonin, our clever little sleep hormone.

    It also helps to ditch the bright, almost radioactive glare of fancy, modern-day clock radios. Instead, go for an old-fashioned alarm clock without a digital display, or try a daylight alarm clock, instead.

    I love my daylight clock, and find that the light starts with a beautiful, deep amber hue and gradually gets brighter to replicate dawn at a pre-set time. There are versions that include a sunset and recordings of waves, tones or music to wake you up. So, instead of waking up to the horrific blare of an alarm in the dark, you wake up gently to a warm, summer's glow. Doesn't that sound better...?

10. Finally, be consistent with your plan. Try to stick with it nine times out of ten, but don't stress out if you miss on a few days. Life happens!

I hope that I've convinced you that making time for beauty sleep really is good for you!

In fact, sleep really is your body's best friend so, if you go to bed late, don't set your clock to get up early for that morning exercise session – it will only be counter-productive.

   If you are lacking sleep, the last thing that your body needs is a grueling session at the gym. Tiredness can actually force the body into preservation mode, meaning it will start storing fuel. What this means for you is that you may not be burning calories while you exercise but, instead, clinging on to them and storing them away.

Stress can be positive

"Stress is like spice - in the right proportion it enhances the flavour of a dish. Too little produces a bland, dull meal; too much may choke you."
– Donald Tubesing

We all know that too much stress is bad for us, but there's a flipside, too – having no stress in our lives can also have a negative impact. Of course, we can't avoid stressful situations, and we all suffer from it in some shape or form, but by understanding how to transform it into a positive experience can change the effect stress has on your body.

   The thing is, good stress gives us that burning fire to go out and achieve and improve the quality of our lives. It can be the push to grow and develop your career, ask for a raise, or book a holiday. Each of our major life events, such as starting a new relationship, getting married, moving house and applying for a new job, can carry an element of stress, too!

Without any stress, there is the potential to become bored and lack motivation.

Stress and your Survival

The problem comes when we are under constant stress. This can raise the risk of all kinds of health problems and put our bodies into 'fight or flight' mode. In emergency situations, your body reacts like there's a rhino about to charge you down and releases a sudden burst of energy.

One of the hormones the body releases under stress is cortisol, a steroid hormone. It's produced by the adrenal glands and, in survival mode, cortisol can be a lifesaver. It works to speed up the heart and pushes blood to the muscles for that extra, all-important burst of energy.

However, the stress we experience in modern-day life doesn't usually call for us to charge away from a wild predator! Instead, workload or finances are the biggest triggers.

When we experience long-term, low-level stress, the body continuously releases cortisol. These ongoing raised levels can lead to inflammation, which we now know can cause all sorts of diseases and symptoms.

Stress and Digestion

What you probably don't know is that stress overload can impact the stomach wall, and this triggers a cataclysm of changes that can affect your health. Around 95 percent of our serotonin levels are produced here, and stressful situations lead to the drying out of the intestinal tract. This creates reactions that flatten down the villi, the little tentacles that absorb our food and nutrients.

As a result, toxins can seep through the cell wall and into the lymph system, creating congestion, tiredness, joint pain, skin breakouts, rashes, allergies and hypersensitivity.

Stress Busting Tips

Meditation and mindfulness can put you back in control of your brain and help you to deal with stressful situations.

There are many books and apps that can teach you all about these wonderful practices, but I swear by this 10 to 15 minute technique, which will help you to find some inner peace and balance.

Are you ready?

- Sit with your eyes closed and turn your attention to your breathing
- Focus on each breath, in and out
- Slowly and deeply, breathe in and out through the nostrils
- Try to concentrate on your breath, and exclude other thoughts
- If your mind wanders, simply bring it back to your breathing

Practice this for just a few minutes a day and you'll soon find that your technique will get much better, and your state of mind will improve, too.

A Quick Technique for De-Stressing

I know that we can all suffer from stress at some point in our lives – we can't escape it. Yet, there's a lot you can do to help your body to relax a little. Here is one of my favourite techniques for de-stressing:

- Sit down with feet firmly planted on the floor
- Close your mouth and breathe in deeply to the count of four
- Hold your breath to the count of seven
- Breathe out firmly through an open mouth, to the count of eight
- Repeat four times

Now, don't you feel better...?

Our Secrets To Natural Beauty

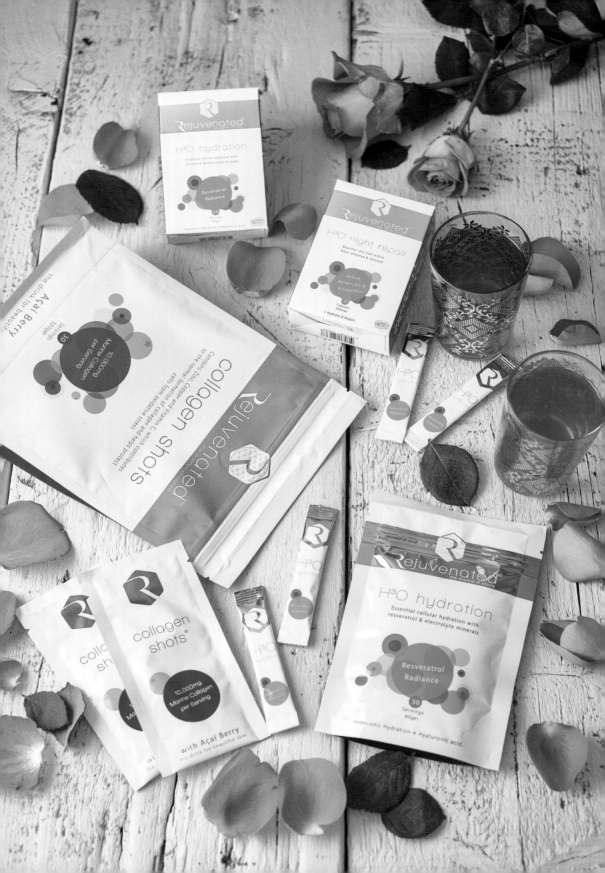

How the Rejuvenated Products Support The Youth Plan

So, now we've armed you with all that knowledge, you're almost ready to start your journey to becoming a healthier, happier, more beautiful and radiant you.

Our Rejuvenated programme is truly unique because we take the perfect sprinkle of nutritious foods and combine it with your lifestyle to help you to appear more youthful. Yet, even though challenging your current diet and lifestyle can bring you boundless energy, glowing skin and that lean body you've always wanted, we can go one step further.

The Rejuvenated products are the result of years and years of research, and we are incredibly proud of them. All along, I wanted to create multi-tasking, 'beauty from within' supplements, which are designed to boost your body from top-to-toe. Brimming with goodness, every product will bring you noticeable results, but when you weave all of them into your life...well, that's when the magic happens!

Each of the products within the Rejuvenated range can boost both inner health and outer beauty, all while delivering long-term solutions and benefits. What's more, they're totally natural, and come without added sugars, fillers or artificial sweeteners. Plus, with the exception of Collagen Shots and Veggiecol, all products are suitable for vegans, while Veggiecol is also suitable for vegetarians.

Collagen Shots® is our hero product! A hydrolysed marine collagen drink, it's also multi award-winning, and packs an almighty youth-boosting punch – it contains 10,000mg of collagen per serving.

Our formula was created to include the highest clinically tested amount of amino acid peptides, which our bodies use to stimulate the production of fibroblasts and collagen.

In addition to that, we also added the 'superfood' acai berry, which contains all sorts of wonderful amino acids, peptides, essential fatty acids, vitamins and minerals. Drinking Collagen Shots will also mean you enjoy plenty of the fountain of youth, Hyaluronic Acid, which attracts and retains up to 1,000 times its own weight in water. This makes a handy cushion between cells to keep skin looking smooth and plump.

Finally, Collagen Shots is full of the minerals copper and zinc to support healthy DNA and protect from oxidative stress, as well as immune-boosting Vitamin C, which contributes to the formation of collagen.

Don't believe us? See what our customers have to say!

"You will see more results in your skin with Collagen Shots than any skin potion I can think of." – *Glynis Barber, actress and co-author of the In-sync Diet*

Next up in our stellar line-up is **H3O Hydration®**, a revolutionary drink which fills the body with all the minerals and ions needed to support hydration.

Every time you sip on H30, you'll receive a beauty-boosting dose of that miraculous hyaluronic acid for cell hydration. You see, this conditioning drink promotes healthy, luminous-looking skin and, by keeping cells hydrated, it keeps them operating at their highest level. This even means that you'll feel less sluggish, and will quickly see a huge improvement in your complexion.

As well as all of this, you can also expect to find:

- Ionic electrolyte minerals to transfer water and nutrients into the blood stream, promoting cellular fluid balance
- Super-charged ingredients, including ionic electrolyte minerals
- A hefty dose of the potent Trans-Resveratrol. This powerful antioxidant is derived from grapes, and helps to protect against ageing free radical attacks
- Hyaluronic acid to cushion the tissue in between the cells
- The water-soluble plant fibre inulin
- Antioxidant Vitamin C

"I recommend all my customers drink H3O Hydration, it boosts hydration levels throughout the whole body for health and beauty." – *Gloria Parfitt, Nutritional Therapist*

H3O Night Repair. This is one tablet with extra va va voom. Our H30 Night Repair is an amazingly potent skin antioxidant, with super hydration. In fact, it wages a multi-pronged attack on the ravages wrought by dehydration – all while you're sleeping and resting. Yet, impressively, it even helps to protect your skin from the sun the next day.

Each little tablet contains:

1. Super hydrating and anti-ageing Hyaluronic Acid
2. Ionic minerals (potassium chloride, magnesium chloride, calcium lactate and sodium citrate) to optimise cellular metabolism and flush out toxins
3. A cocktail of vitamins (A, B, C, D and E) to protect against free radicals, support the immune system and accelerate metabolic function

4. Astaxanthin – a unique source of super-potent sea algae with many, many more times the antioxidant power of vitamin C, beta carotene or green tea. This protects against skin-ageing environmental aggressors
5. Astragulus – a herb believed to increase the production of telomerase (the enzyme integral to the cellular division process)

"If beauty sleep came in a packet it would look a lot like this." *– Get the Gloss*

Veggiecol® is the first vegetarian-friendly natural collagen supplement. It comes in a handy capsule and uses a unique, patented egg extract, with over 500 active ingredients.

We've added the same super active ingredients that are hiding within Collagen Shots, including Hyaluronic Acid, super fruit acai berry, Vitamin C, Vitamin B (niacin), copper and zinc. This means you see all the beauty-loving benefits of our traditional Collagen Shots in a handy, vegetarian-friendly form.

"A really good nutriceutical supplement 'super-charges' your high-end serum – in fact if you're not taking one (and live in a city) you're almost doing your skin a disservice. New Veggicol capsules, from the makers of the hugely successful Collagen Shots, are a clever, handbag-friendly vegetarian alternative to marine collagen – gluten-free, they're packed with skin-quenching hyaluronic acid, 'de-wrinkling' glucosamine and chondroitin and antioxidant superhero acai berry and a nice added extra is the beauty boost they'll give your hair and nails, too" *– Beauty Shortlist Award team*

The role Rejuvenated plays in boosting your Natural Moisture Factor:

As you can see, these products work their magic from the inside, out. Yet, they also have a huge impact on the superficial layers of the skin.

Our **Natural Moisturising Factor**, or **NMF**, is a collection of water-soluble compounds that are only found in the outer layer of the skin. This outer layer, otherwise known as the stratum corneum, was always thought to be biologically dead. However, we now know that this isn't quite true. Instead, it has a strange, dynamic structure where enzymes remain active, but need water to perform their duties.

The role of the NMF is to support skin hydration so that our superficial layer can stay resilient, while enzymes get to work on breaking down dead skin. This reveals fresher, healthier skin below.

Our NMF is high in amino acids and inorganic minerals such as chlorides, phosphates, sodium, potassium, calcium and magnesium. These work together like a special skin magnet, attracting water from the atmosphere and, in turn, creating firmer, more hydrated skin.

By combining our powerful trio of Collagen Shots, H3O Hydration and H3O Night Repair, you'll provide full support to the NMF, with plenty of amino acid proteins and minerals.

Rejuvenated Protein Smoothie is another of our powerful body-loving products. It's a delicious, vegan pea protein drink, which we created for both fitness lovers and health enthusiasts to help them lose weight and boost strength.

Unlike many protein brands on the market, each drink contains 100 percent naturally-active ingredients. Sipping on it pre- or post-workout will help to send muscle-firming amino acids surging through the body, and can even balance out blood sugar levels.

This delicious drink also contains the fashionable ingredient inulin, which is found in plants and is a super-concentrated form of starch. However, most impressively, inulin works to counteract visceral fat hidden around the heart and other organs, the most dangerous kind of fat to our health.

Each Rejuvenated Protein Smoothie is also rich in key muscle-firming amino acids, and can help to keep you feeling fuller for longer, all while building long, lean muscles.

Providing a hefty 21 grams of pea protein, it's the easy, delicious way to introduce more protein into your diet. It can also support healthy blood sugar levels, supercharge the immune system, boost hormone production and help with weight control.

We use organic pea protein, it is incredibly effective at building lean tissue (the thing that gives you beautiful, long muscles). This is because it's rich in branch chain amino acids and compounds that help to delay fatigue during exercise.

Pea protein really delivers, and is a superior alternative to dairy, soy and whey-based products. Just check out these results if you remain unconvinced:

1. Pea protein naturally reduces appetite, while glucommanan fibre from the konjac plant gently swells in the stomach to keep you feeling fuller for longer
2. Inulin counteracts visceral fat and promotes natural intestinal health, all while regulating blood sugar levels
3. Green tea containing polyphenols can gently induce thermogenesis and stimulate fat oxidation
4. Flaxseed is loaded with body-loving Omega-3 for skin and cellular health

Protein Soup. Our brand-new, delicious and organic pea protein soup is full of tasty, freeze-dried vegetables and herbs, as well as antioxidants, vitamins, minerals, and fibre. It counts as one of your five-a-day, and is a real hug in a mug!

Unlike most other ready soups on the market, ours is pretty special. It contains that wondrous organic pea protein, as well as glucomannan fibre, Omega-3 and super potent vegetables. Combine these incredible ingredients, and it's no wonder that we're proud of this instant soup. It's the perfect nourishing snack or meal accompaniment, and is ready in just seconds to power you through your day!

As you may already know, pea protein is rich in key muscle-firming amino acids (lysine, arginine, glutamine) and branched-chain amino acids (luecine, isoleucine, valine). Thanks to these little miracles, Protein Soup helps you to stay fuller for longer, as well as supporting beautiful skin and building that firm, lean muscle that we all desire. It's an essential for anyone looking for healthy weight loss, or for those of us who simply want a comforting, delicious soup to sip on.

Beauty Cake® is one of my favourite products. After all, who wouldn't love a beauty-boosting cake? It is a delicious protein-based cake designed to nourish from within. Crafted with mouth-watering ingredients, this is one treat you'll never need to feel guilty about.

While Beauty Cake is designed to nourish the skin, it also delivers a high-protein alternative to sugary snacks, and is one of our Rejuvenated range of products to promote healthy weight loss and blood sugar levels:

Aliol® is a clever capsule which can give you a powerful boost of vegan-friendly Omega-3 oil from plant-based algae.

Omega-3 is vital for every single cell in our body, even though we can't create it naturally. The most potent form of Omega-3 comes from fish oils, which is why you're told to load your plates with oily fish, or take a capsule form. Of course, this is fine, but what about vegans? As well as that, fish oil capsules leave a pretty nasty taste in the mouth, and can cause bad breath!

Aliol is a powerhouse of plant-based Omega-3 which keeps the heart strong and supports brain health. It is 100 percent plant-based and comes from the algae that fish actually feed on, meaning it's the dream supplement for all sorts of diets, including vegetarians and vegans.

Each precious capsule contains high amounts of DHA (docosahexaenoic acid), which is an environmentally-friendly Omega-3 fatty acid. Clinical research shows that DHA offers incredible health benefits for brain heart and skin health.

Finally, **Re-set** is a naturally-active health food supplement that we created for those looking to lose weight healthily. Its potent cocktail of ingredients work to boost cellular health, stabilise blood sugar levels and our metabolism, all while promoting lean and healthy tissue for total, top-to-toe well-being.

"I love Re-set. It helps to balance my sugar levels so that I don't get snack attacks during the day" – Sandra Cooke, Celebrity make up artist

Our whole range has been formulated to support and supplement the Rejuvenated Lifestyle programme. You can use the programme on its own, or mix and match with whichever products you fancy. See us as your very own beauty-based pick and mix!

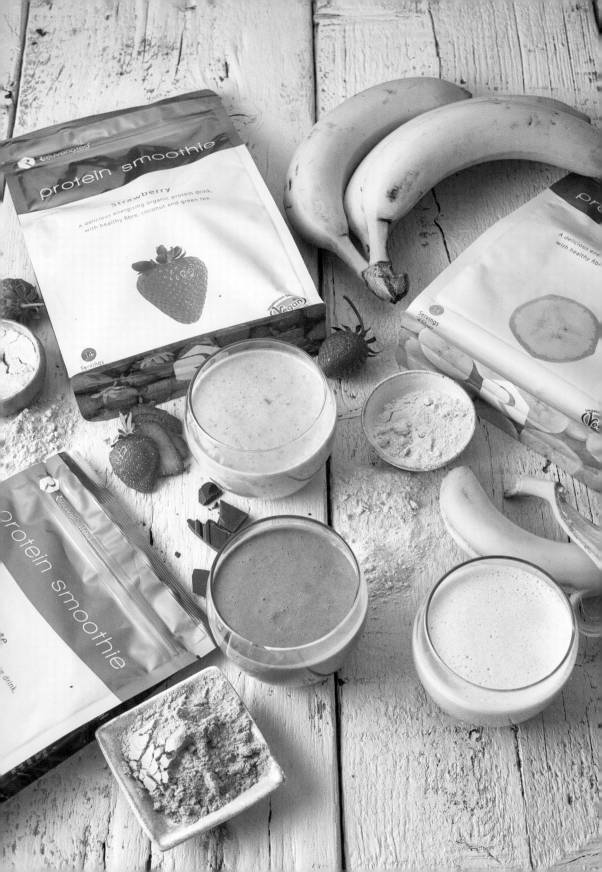

The Best Project You Will Ever Work On Is You

THE ULTIMATE PROJECT – YOU

Trust me when I say that I've been sitting exactly where you are right now, and I know that it's not always easy to dive head-first into a new regime.

Yet, we can do this together – you can do this – and I guarantee that you will soon feel better and healthier than ever before; the best project you will ever work on is you.

How do you want to feel in 30 days' time?

In this first week, we are going to focus on making some diet and food changes to give you more vitality, and to get your body glowing from head-to-toe.

It helps to set yourself goals, and one of the tricks I like to use is to visualise myself in 30 days' time – take a couple of moments to close your eyes and picture it, too. What's happened in the 30 days?

- I have more energy
- I'm happy
- I'm fitter
- I've lost...lbs
- I'm wearing...

Write down below what you can see, but don't set your goals too high. Instead, it helps to create ones that you can achieve and celebrate, no matter how small.

In 30 days' time, I...

At the end of this programme, you will be able to live your life to the full and forget your age. Trust me when I say that youth and beauty are ageless.

Sometimes, you will fall short, but don't worry – we all do, and life happens! Yet, whatever the ups and downs, I promise that Rejuvenated will set you on a new path, a fresh new journey, and you'll soon be shining and revealing the beautiful person that you are.

Your First Week

GREAT NUTRITION MADE EASY

Now that we've come this far, it's time to roll up those sleeves and get started!

I know that there are very few people who have hours to spare to slave away in the kitchen. With this in mind, we've kept most of the recipes quite simple so that you can cook up delicious, mouth-watering food in no time at all.

If you're conscious of budget, then don't fret. We've also stayed mindful of the cost, helping you to use up the ingredients in your fridge and cupboards wherever possible.

If you do find yourself loving our food and meal ideas, then take some time to scroll through our website for more inspiration. There, you'll find many more recipes, including some from our brand ambassadors and friends. We always love to hear about your favourites, and welcome any that you think we should add to the site!

As well as delicious, nourishing foods, we also like to arm ourselves (and our bodies) with our Rejuvenated products. When taken alongside a healthy, balanced diet, they can help you to achieve your goals, and give you some extra options to reach for throughout the day. In fact, they're ideal for enjoying when you're on the go, or simply too busy to prepare food.

I particularly love taking five minutes to enjoy a delicious glass of Rejuvenated Protein Smoothie mid-afternoon. This is a high-quality pea protein drink packed with healthy Omega-3s, as well as green tea and glucomannan fibre to keep you feeling full and to balance out healthy cholesterol levels.

It comes in three flavours and is quick, nutritious and satisfying. Plus, you can have an experiment and drink it however you fancy – mix it with water or nut milk, add in spoonfuls of almond butter or oats, or even add fruit and vegetables to suit your taste.

However, a quick word to the wise: don't substitute more than one meal and one snack per day. Real, whole foods will nourish your body and your skin in every possible way!

Now, here's your handy meal plan to set aside and keep. Enjoy, and eat up with a smile!

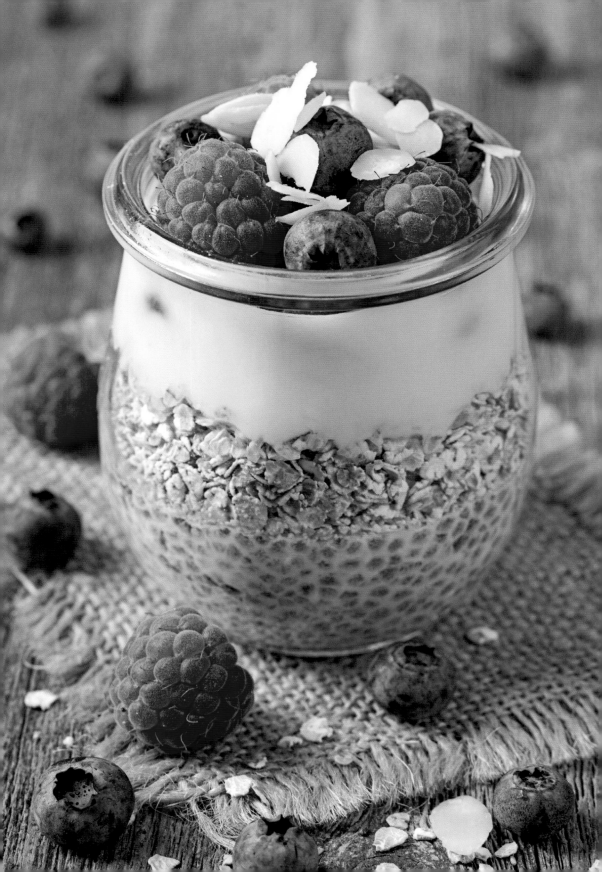

BREAKFAST

Try one of these delicious meals first thing:

- Rejuvenated Protein Smoothie

- Two Egg Omelette – eggs are an excellent source of protein, Vitamin B, lecithin (for skin) and choline for energy

- Egg Muffins – These sweet little mini omelettes are baked in a muffin tin, and can be kept in the fridge for a tasty, protein-rich snack

- Poached or Grilled Salmon with Scrambled Eggs and Spinach

- Mushroom and Tomato Frittata

- Overnight Oats (this is as easy as soaking oats in water or nut milk overnight, then topping with berries, seeds and nuts the next day)

- Porridge with Seeds, Nuts and Berries

- Chia Pudding

- Poached Plums with Yogurt and Sprinkled Nuts

- Roasted Beetroot with Goat's Cheese

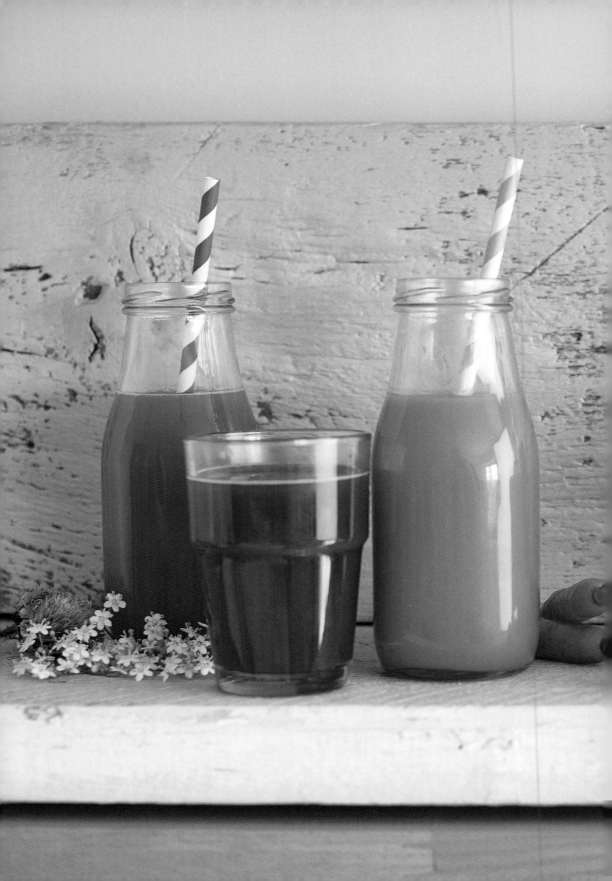

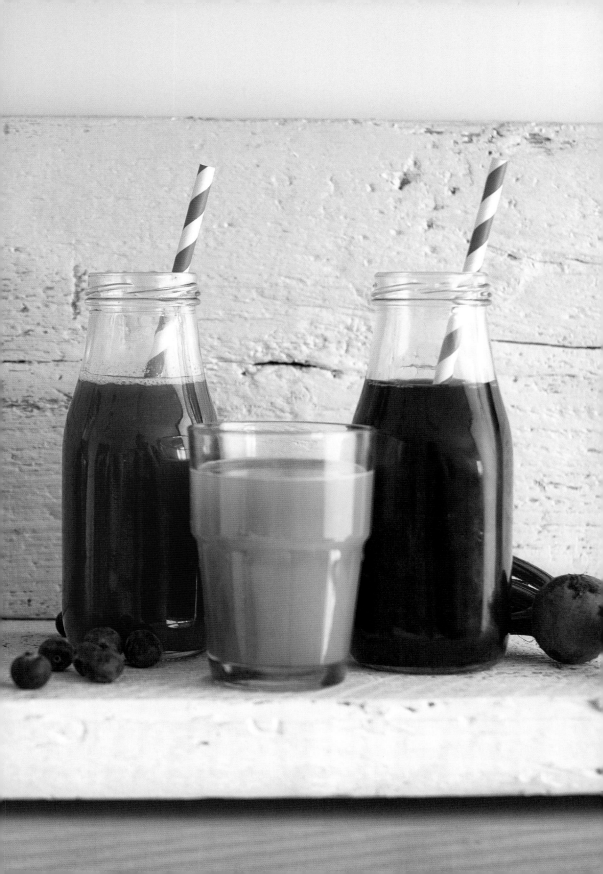

Juices And Drinks

Put down the pre-packaged orange juice! Instead, set yourself a new challenge and try making your own juices, combining both fruit and veggies to keep blood sugar levels stable. As an added tip, I find that adding ginger and apple tends to make everything taste delicious!

If you fancy an extra boost, you can always combine your homemade juices with Protein Smoothie to make a super shake. However, remember that avocado and banana don't juice, so if you want to add these, then blend them in afterwards.

Once you've started juicing, you'll soon find your own favourites by experimenting with different combinations – be adventurous and don't be afraid! Just dust off that juicer or blender, raid your fridge and go for it!

However, if you do want a little guidance, then here are some of my favourites to start you off.

Vitality Juice –

Ingredients:
- Two beetroot
- Two carrots
- 1cm cube ginger, peeled
- One apple

Toss all ingredients into your juicer for the perfect boost to your energy levels. Beetroot is a nutritional powerhouse and an energiser – it dilates and strengthens blood vessels to give increased blood flow for stamina, and even helps to reduce blood pressure and nourishes the brain. Carrots and ginger add to this effect, while apples are excellent anti-inflammatories.

Berry Booster for Antioxidant Protection –

Ingredients:
- Two apples
- Handful black seedless grapes
- Handful pitted black cherries
- Handful blueberries
- One capsule Aliol or flaxseed oil

Juice the apples, then pour into a blender along with the dark fruits (a juicer will remove the nutritious, fibrous skins from the berries and grapes) and blitz, popping in either the contents of an Aliol capsule or or ½ a tablespoon of flaxseed oil for omega-3 benefits.

The Anti-Ager –

Ingredients:
- ½ mango
- Four carrots
- 1cm cube ginger, peeled

Beta carotene is a skin-loving antioxidant that gives mangoes and carrots their bright and beautiful orange colour. The human body converts beta carotene into Vitamin A, which is a powerful anti-ager for both the skin and our immune system. Meanwhile, marvelous mangoes have high levels of magnesium and phenolic acid which help to calm the central nervous system to destress. Simply make this by juicing all ingredients, then drinking and enjoying!

The Heart Booster –

Ingredients:
- 1 head of celery
- 2 beetroot
- 1 large apple

It's widely accepted that beetroot and celery can help to reduce blood pressure levels, why not combine the two with something like apple or carrot.

Cool, Calm Cucumber for Sensitised Skin –

Ingredients:
- One apple
- ¼ of a cucumber
- Two sticks celery
- One kiwi
- 1cm cube ginger, peeled
- ½ avocado

Green vegetables can work wonders at calming inflamed and sensitive skin. Cooling cucumber is miraculous for detoxification, as is celery, while kiwi is packed with Vitamin C and ginger is calming. Meanwhile, creamy avocado is full of healthy fats to nourish the skin and can help with conditions such as rosacea, eczema and psoriasis. To make this cooling drink, juice all of the ingredients, apart from the avocado, then add to a blender along with the avocado, before blitzing smooth.

When you really can't wait until dinner

If you find yourself hungry mid-morning or afternoon, then you don't need to raid the biscuit tin, or dash for the vending machine. Try these simple snacks for happier, healthier snacking, always aiming to include protein, which will keep you fuller for longer.

Here are some of my go-to snacks for when those munchies suddenly strike...

- Rejuvenated Protein Smoothie

- Our Protein Soup is a warming and nourishing hug in a mug, and is formulated with organic pea protein

- Beautycake® is our delicious and nutritious protein cake, and has been created for maximum nourishment with pumpkin seed protein

- A handful of olives

- Avocado mash on two rice cakes or gluten-free oat cakes

- Chickpea salad

- A small handful of brazil nuts (maximum seven per day), walnuts, hazelnuts or almonds

- 4oz of cottage cheese

- Smoked salmon with two rice cakes or gluten-free oatcakes

- A boiled egg

- Small serving of Greek salad*

- 2oz of quinoa, combined with chopped onion, one tomato and two chopped olives

- Roasted butterbeans with olive oil, dried sage and a sprinkling of salt and black pepper

- 4oz portion of chicken, lean beef or salmon

- Berries and Greek yogurt

recipes for this dishes appear later on in the book

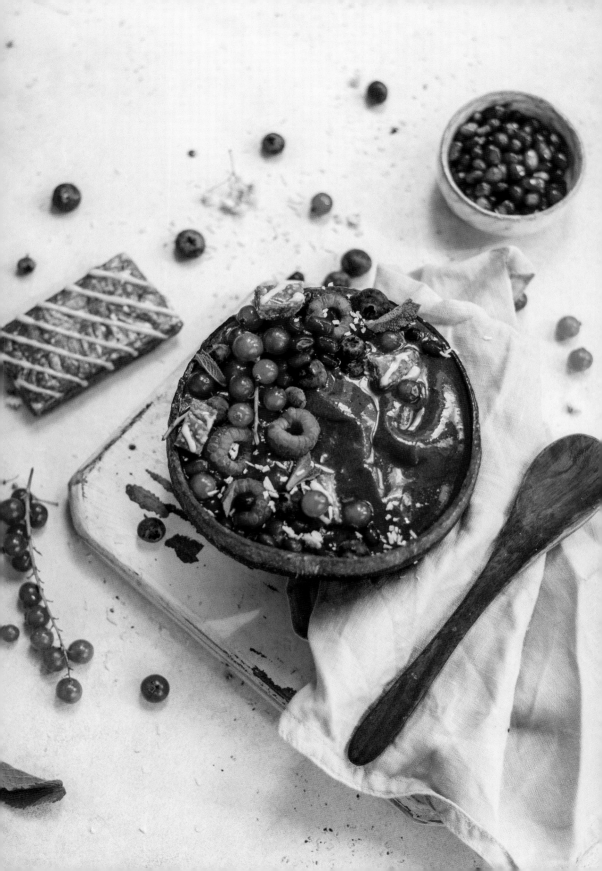

MENUS

How to Get the Best From Our Menus

To stay as healthy and as energized as possible, I find that it helps to get organised at the weekend and plan for the week ahead. I try to set aside a couple of hours on a Sunday afternoon to make my snacks and meals for the next few days. However, healthy eating should fit around your lifestyle.

If you can find meal times overwhelming, then please see the Youth Plan as a little kickstarter, something to guide you through those first few days and even weeks.

We're giving you a helping hand with our shopping list, but remember that this is only a guide for lunches and dinners – you'll need to think about what you will want for snacks and, which is where many of us fall down!

However, now that you're ready to begin, read on, enjoy and feel inspired! The menus and recipes on the following pages are packed with our favourite Youth Plan foods to nourish and reveal your most youthful, beautiful you.

In the meantime, try to remember these simple tips to help you on your way:

- When eating protein, a serving should be around the size of your palm. Pile the rest of your plate high with delicious green leaves and veggies.

- In the first week, you'll be investing in some store foods which should last you for the whole month. You can buy meat and fish ready-frozen in large packs for the month ahead, ready to defrost for meals.

- Use fresh herbs wherever possible as these will flavour your foods and make your meals sing. If you find it expensive, then buying a plant should provide you with enough leaves for the whole month and much longer, too. If you're starting the Youth Plan programme in spring or summer, then try planting salad, spinach and beet leaves in a seed tray, ready to harvest in just four weeks' time.

Of course, please try to remember that this plan has been designed to be flexible, and the meals can be changed around to fit in with your likes and lifestyle. We know that everyone is different, especially when it comes to tastebuds!

I find that it also helps to mix up the proteins according to what your local markets have in supply. For salads, vegetables and stir fries, you could also simply use whatever you have in your fridge – these are just guidelines to follow.

Now, let's get started!

First up, let's pick your breakfasts and snacks from the suggested lists. And remember, if you're feeling rushed or uninspired, one meal per day can be substituted with Rejuvenated's Protein Smoothie Drink or Protein Soup. Take one Re-set tablet with breakfast and lunch.

WEEK ONE MENUS:

	Breakfast	Lunch	Dinner
Mon	Protein Smoothie	Super Green Quinoa* and Herb Green Leaf Salad	Thai Prawns* and Rejuvenated Salad*
Tue	Protein Smoothie	Roast Carrot and Garlic Soup*	Fillet of Salmon, Quinoa & Roast Vegetables*
Wed	Protein Smoothie	Smoked Salmon, Black Olives, half an Avocado and Green Salad	Chicken Breast & Stir Fry Vegetables of Choice
Thu	Protein Smoothie	Coconut and Butternut Squash Soup*	Cod or Haddock with Sweet Potato & Butternut Squash Mash, Green Beans and Grilled Tomato
Fri	Protein Smoothie	Leftovers of either soup made earlier in the week	Two Egg Omelette with Green Leaves, Olives and Pine Nuts
Sat	Protein Smoothie	Baked Sweet Potato, Beetroot, Salad Leaves, Onion, Tomato & Peas	Roast Chicken with Roast Vegetables and Peas
Sun	Protein Smoothie	Salad Niçoise*	Lamb Steak, Baked Sweet Potato and Rejuvenated Salad*

recipes for these dishes appear later on in the book

And here's that handy shopping list to keep in your purse, or to stick to your fridge:

Protein -

One pack of prawns
Two chicken portions
One tuna steak/tin of tuna
Two salmon fillets
One cod

Fruit & Vegetables -

One bag of carrots
One butternut squash
One small red cabbage
One bag of red onions
Two avocados
Two red peppers
Two courgettes
12 tomatoes
One pack of green beans
Three bulbs of garlic
Green leaves of choice (spinach/kale/Swiss chard, pak choi, watercress)
Small piece of ginger root
Optional fresh parsley
Two lemons or limes
Alfalfa sprouts, if available

Pantry -

Six eggs
Packet of quinoa
Bouillon
Tamari
Walnuts
Olives
Pumpkin seeds
Tin of coconut milk
Grape seed oil, for cooking
Olive oil, for salads
Turmeric
Chilli flakes
Ground coriander
Pumpkin seeds

Freezer -

Bag of frozen peas

Rejuvenated task - Take the 7-day hydration challenge

Now that we're getting into the swing of things, let's turn our heads to upping our intake of water.

For me, it helps to start each day by gulping down a refreshing glass of water, and by keeping a handy water bottle on my desk or close by. To really reap the rewards, try adding in a sprinkling of H3O Hydration to enhance the effects and to help balance fluid levels.

I also find that it helps to make notes in my Rejuvenated diary. You could try jotting down:

- How do you feel when you are more hydrated?
- Do you have more energy?
- Do your eyes look brighter?
- How's your concentration level?

Doesn't that feel better?

Now that you're feeling hydrated and your skin is plumped up and dewy fresh, here's your **Week 2 Meal Plan:**

WEEK TWO MENUS:

	Breakfast	Lunch	Dinner
Mon	Protein Smoothie	Goats Cheese with Beetroot*, Salad Leaves. Tomato and Onion	Salmon and Puy lentils with Rejuvenated Salad *and Dressing of your choice
Tue	Protein Smoothie	Beetroot Soup* Topped with Goat's Cheese and Parsley	Prawns and Cashew Stir Fry*
Wed	Protein Smoothie	Smoked Salmon and half an Avocado on Rice Cakes	Two Egg Omelette with Salad and Remaining Avocado

Thu	Protein Smoothie	Roast Carrot Soup*	Chicken, Quinoa and Roast Vegetables*
Fri	Protein Smoothie	Chicken and Spinach Salad	Lean Lamb or Chickpea Burgers*
Sat	Protein Smoothie	Roast Carrot Soup*	Pearl Barley and Mushroom Supper*
Sun	Protein Smoothie	Super Green Quinoa*	Salmon with Sweet Potato and Roast Vegetables

recipes for these dishes appear later on in the book

And, of course, here's that fail-safe shopping list to help keep you on-track this week:

For the Fridge -
Prawns
Minced, lean lamb
Salmon fillet
Goat's cheese
Two portions of chicken

Mange tout
Two red peppers
Two courgettes
Green leaves
(see last week's selection for ideas)
Spinach
Alfalfa sprouts, if available

Fruit & Vegetables -
One pack of raw beetroot
Tomatoes
Green leaves
One bag of carrots
One bag of onions
Avocado
One punnet of mushrooms
One bag of sweet potatoes

Pantry -
One carton or tin of chopped tomatoes
Puy lentils
Quinoa
Pearl Barley
Cashew nuts
Tin of chickpeas

Exercise not only changes your body.
It changes your mind, your attitude and your mood.

WEEK THREE MENUS:

	Breakfast	Lunch	Dinner
Mon	Protein Smoothie	Guacamole and Rice or Oat Cakes	White Fish with Pistachio Pesto* and Salad of Choice
Tue	Protein Smoothie	Coconut and Butternut Squash Soup*	Chick Pea Burgers* and Roast Vegetables
Wed	Protein Smoothie	Two Egg Omelette with Mushrooms and Spinach	White Fish with Quinoa and Roast Vegetables
Thu	Protein Smoothie	Coconut and Butternut Squash Soup*	Dinner Thai Prawns* and Stir Fry
Fri	Protein Smoothie	Poached Eggs and Ratatouille*	Mackerel and Beetroot Salad*
Sat	Protein Smoothie	Protein of choice and Rejuvenated Salad*	Pearl Barley and Mushroom Supper*
Sun	Protein Smoothie	Alfredo's Salad*	Herb Chicken* and Roast Vegetables

recipes for these dishes appear later on in the book

And here's that handy shopping list to keep in your purse, or to stick to your fridge:

Protein –

Four eggs
Two white fish
One pack of prawns
One mackerel
Two chicken portions

Fruit & Vegetables –

Two avocados
Green leaves
Coriander
One pack of raw beetroot
One punnet of mushrooms
Butternut squash
Two red peppers
Two courgettes
One pack of tomatoes
One pack of stir fry veg
Two onions
Spinach
Four garlic cloves
One red chilli or chilli flakes

Pantry –

Pistachio nuts
Quinoa
Tin of chopped tomatoes
Oat cakes
Olive oil
Tin of coconut milk
Tin of chickpeas
Tin of tuna
Mixed herbs
Pearl barley

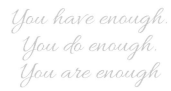

You have enough.
You do enough.
You are enough

Relax . . . . .

Rest and relaxation

When we rest our energy is restored, you don't always need to be getting things done. It's absolutely necessary and perfectly ok to stop, rest and breath.

Whether it's a little yoga, meditation, sleep or mindfulness, whatever allows you to let go of tension and become renewed.

WEEK FOUR MENUS:

	Breakfast	*Lunch*	*Dinner*
Mon	Protein Smoothie	Two Egg Omelette with half an Avocado and Watercress	Salmon and Rejuvenated Salad* using rest of Avocado
Tue	Protein Smoothie	Chicken Breast and Stir Fry Vegetables of choice	Coconut and Butternut Squash Soup*
Wed	Protein Smoothie	Goat's Cheese Salad*	Thai Prawns* (Meat or Vegetables can be used if desired) and Herb Green Leaf Salad
Thu	Protein Smoothie	Mediterranean Vegetables and Cannellini Mash*	Salmon, Sweet Potato and Roast Vegetables or Salad

Fri	Protein Smoothie	Coconut and Butternut Squash Soup*	Chicken and Sweet Potato with Green Leaf Salad
Sat	Protein Smoothie	Salad Niçoise*	Sweet Potato Omelette* and Green Beans
Sun	Protein Smoothie	Mediterranean Vegetables and Cannellini Mash*	Grilled Lamb Steak, Ratatouille* and Green Salad

*recipes for these dishes appear later on in the book

Shopping list:

Protein -
Six eggs
Two salmon fillets
Two chicken breasts
One tuna steak or tin of tuna
One lamb steak
One pack of prawns

Fruit & Vegetables -
Two avocados
One butternut squash
One bag of onions
One bag of watercress
Two red peppers
One aubergine
One bag of sweet potatos
One bulb of garlic
One pack of green beans
(can be thawed from frozen)
One cucumber

One pack of mushrooms
One bag of stir fry or use other vegetables bought
One bag of salad leaves
Eight tomatoes
Half a red cabbage
One sprig of coriander
One pack of alfalfa sprouts
Non essential
Parsley – for decoration

Pantry -
One 400ml can of coconut milk
One pack of olives
One packet of pearl barley
Tin of cannellini beans

Freezer -
All items can be bought from freezer where appropriate

Recipes

Breakfasts & Omelettes

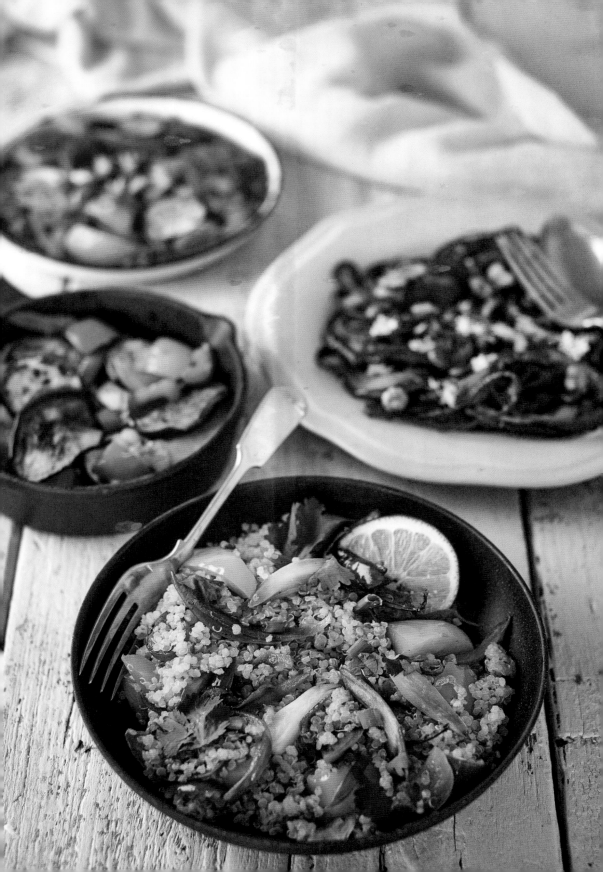

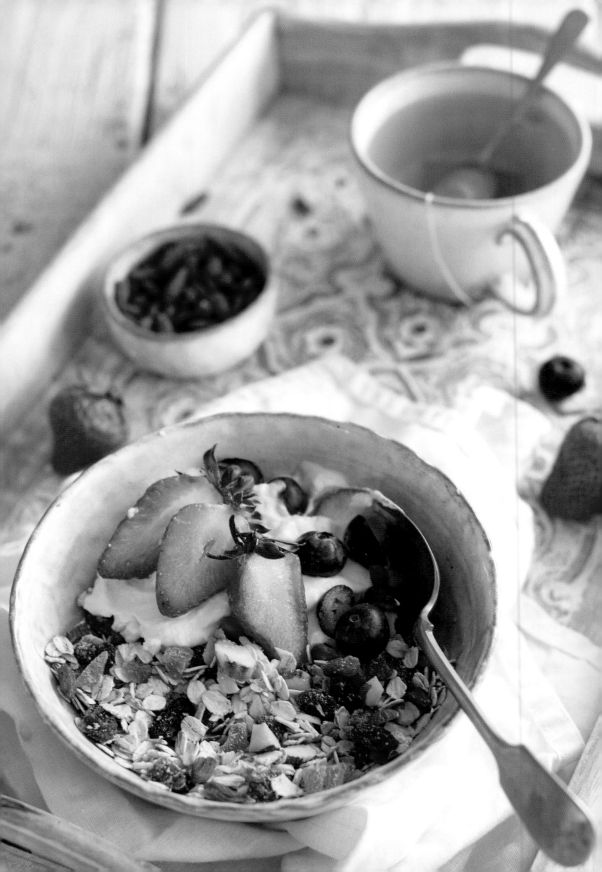

SUPER MUESLI

This is a super-nutritious base for a muesli, full of vitamins, minerals, Omega-3 oils and fibres. You can add your favourite fruits, yogurt, non-dairy milk, whatever you choose to give it a different tweak every day.

Ingredients

Per bowl

2tbsp oats
2 almonds, chopped
2 Brazil nuts chopped
1 apricot, chopped
1tsp sultanas
1tsp flaxseed ground

Method

Mix together the ingredients, then store in an airtight container ready for eating. I like to spoon mine over yoghurt, or serve with nut milk.

Rejuvenated Porridge

This is our favourite winter morning treat. Our daughter Lois brought back the recipe whilst on her travels in Australia. It has just about every vitamin that your body could need. It does take a while to prepare but it's well worth it, I have a drawer that I keep all the key ingredients together in. She shared the recipe with Daniel Sandler and he has been a firm convert ever since.

Ingredients

Per bowl

1tbsp oats
5-6 almonds
2-3 walnuts
1tbsp chia seeds
1tsp sunflower seeds
1tsp pumpkin seeds
Half tbsp cinnamon
Half tbsp coconut oil
Half a banana, sliced
Few blueberries
2-3 strawberries
2tbsp dried goji berries
A sprinkle of desiccated coconut or coconut flakes
2-3tbsp hot water

There are quite a lot of ingredients but this bowl does come together quite quickly and it will keep you full for hours.

Method

• Put the oats, nuts, seeds, cinnamon and coconut oil into the bowl.
• Add the hot water and stir to mix well.
• Top with fruit, goji berries and finally coconut.
Enjoy!

TIP
Vary your toppings according to fruits that are in season.

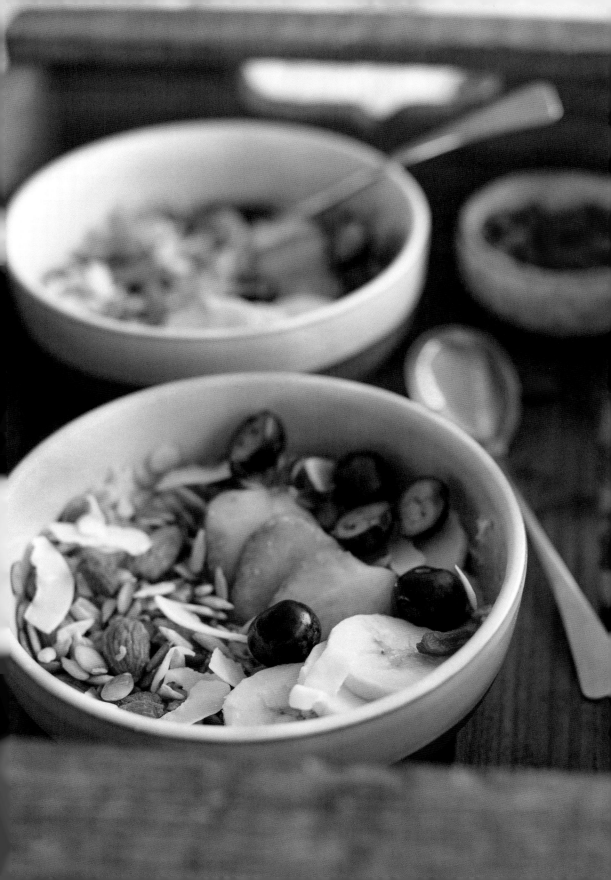

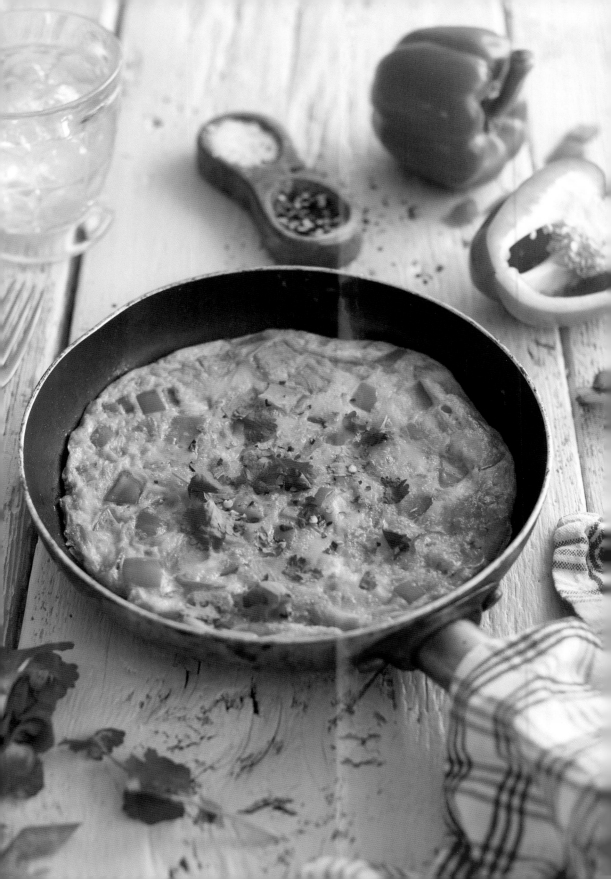

PLAIN OMELETTE

There is nothing to beat an omelette for a healthy quick meal and an easy way to add nourishing protein to your diet. They also contain healthy fats, Vitamin B2, B6, and D and minerals such as selenium, copper, zinc and iron, You can have it plain or add some nutrient boosters as the recipes below.

2 eggs
Splash of non-dairy milk
Salt and black pepper to taste

RED PEPPER & SWEET POTATO OMELETTE

Add a red pepper to load up antioxidants, from carotenoids concentrated in the flesh of the pepper. The range of benefits provided by these colourful pigments include improved immune function, better communication between cells, protection against sun damage, and a diminished risk for several types of cancer.

Ingredients

2 eggs
Splash of non-dairy milk
Half red pepper
1 small sweet potato

Method

- Peel and dice sweet potato – boil until soft.
- Gently fry red pepper – you can use any veg for this.
- Meanwhile, beat eggs, add a splash of milk and seasoning.
- Turn up heat slightly add drained sweet potato and eggs.
- Cook omelette to your liking.

Soups

Carrot & Coriander Soup

This is a healthy twist on a classic soup using yeast free vegetable stock and coconut oil instead of cream. All the delicious taste but super good for you too.

Ingredients

Serves 2

2tsp coconut oil
1 onion, peeled and chopped
2 garlic cloves, peeled and minced
4 carrots, peeled and chopped
400ml yeast-free vegetable stock
Sea salt
Freshly ground black pepper

Method

- Gently soften the onions and garlic by frying in coconut oil on a low heat.
- Add chopped carrots and soften for 3-4 minutes.
- Pour in the vegetable stock and bring to a boil, reducing the heat to a simmer and cooking until the carrots are tender.
- Add coriander, salt and pepper before turning into a blender and blitzing to your desired consistency.
- You may wish to add a little ginger or chilli before blending.

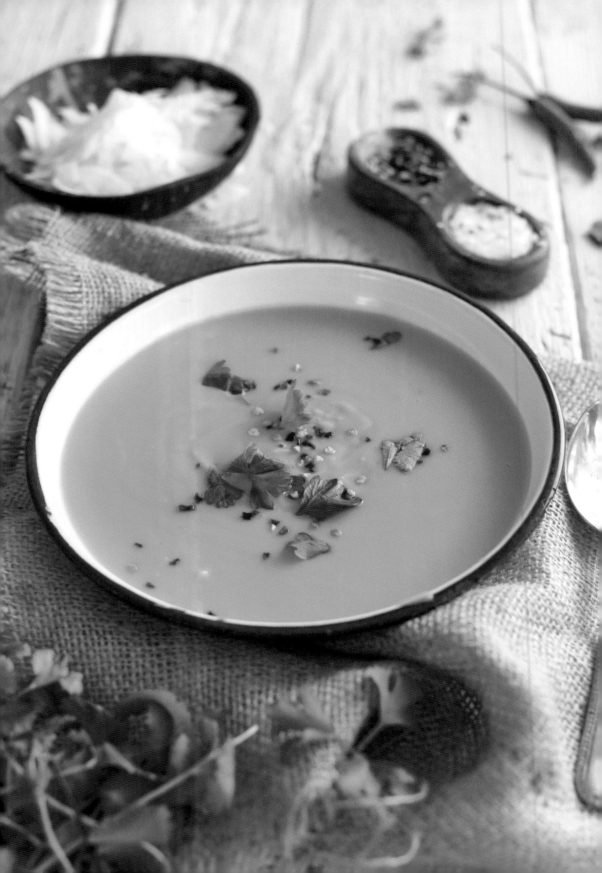

Coconut & Butternut Squash Soup

The coconut milk gives this soup a rich creamy texture. It's perfect for winter evenings but a gorgeous summer treat too. The coconut adds medium chain fatty acids, some of them good fats that actually help you to burn more calories off.

Ingredients

Serves 4

1 400ml can coconut milk
1 butternut squash
1 white onion, chopped
2tbsp coconut or grape seed oil
250ml vegetable stock
Pinch Himalayan salt
Chopped parsley, to serve

Method

- Slice the butternut squash in half, then wrap in foil and roast until soft (around 30 minutes).
- Add the oil to a pan on the hob and heat, before gently frying the onion until softened.
- Pour in the coconut milk, then add the squash and vegetable stock and simmer for 20 minutes.
- Allow to cool slightly, then blend the soup until smooth in a blender before returning to the pan.
- Serve with sprinkled parsley.

TIP
For a variation, try adding a sprinkling of chili flakes to spice things up and chick peas or beans for more protein.

Roast Carrot & Garlic Soup

A delicious soup, packed with so much goodness that it will have you glowing inside and out. Carrots are rich in beta carotene, one of the carotenoids is an orange pigment which gives great health benefits particularly for skin and eye health. While onions and garlic both have healing properties and are believed to be good for heart health and to help protect against cancer.

Ingredients

Serves 3-4

Bag of carrots
2 onions
5 garlic cloves, peeled and minced
1tbsp grape seed oil
Half pint vegetable bouillon

Method

- Wash and peel the carrots, then drizzle with grape seed oil and roast for 10 minutes on a lined baking tray. Add the garlic cloves and continue roasting until the carrots start to crisp at the edges.
- Meanwhile, gently fry onions and prepare the bouillon.
- Once the carrots are cooked, add them to the bouillon mixture and blend smooth. Return to the heat in a saucepan, heating to the desired temperature.

TIP
For a tasty variation, substitute some of the bouillon with chopped tomatoes.

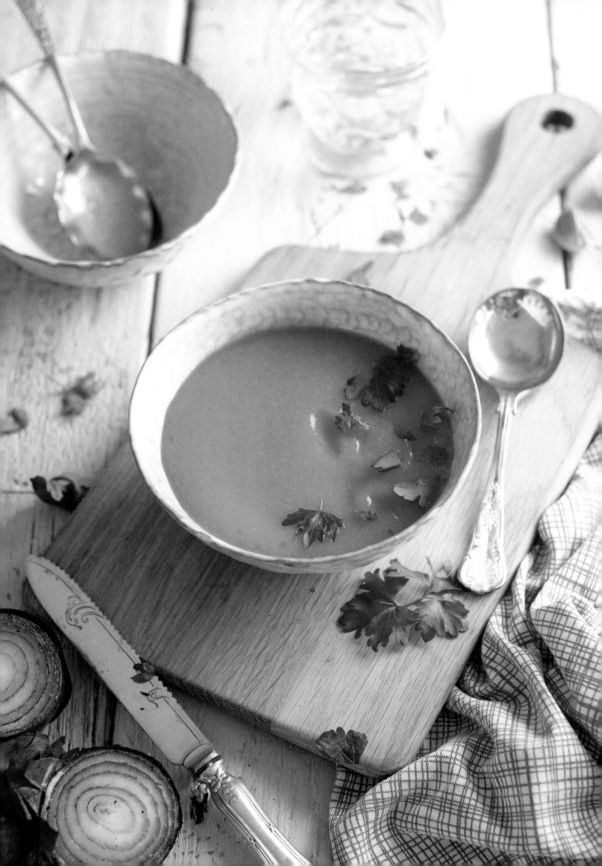

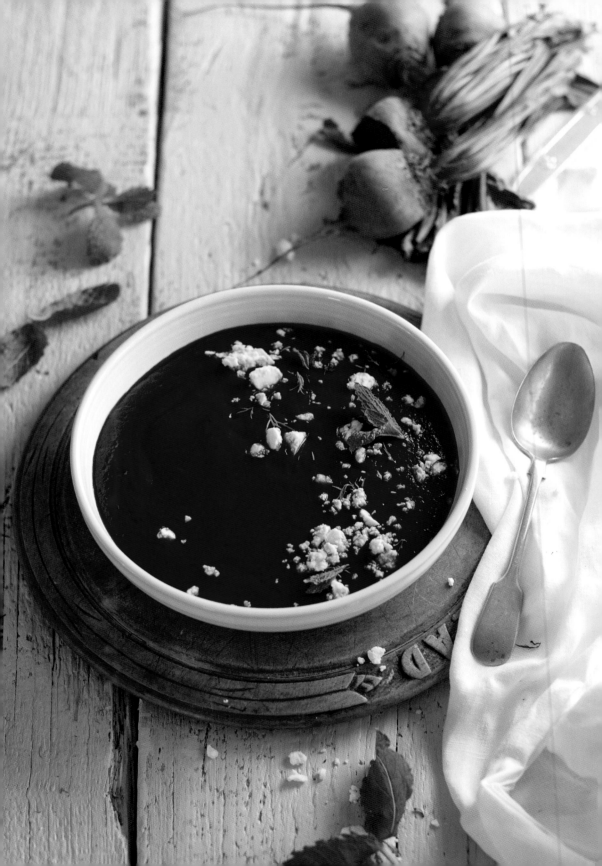

Beetroot Soup with Goat's Cheese & Parsley

We love beetroot and include it in so many different recipes. Beetroots have been one of the most underrated veggies around. They are amazing for the heart and arterial health; they also give an energy boost to power you through the day. If you haven't tried a beetroot soup yet, we'd definitely recommend that you give it a go. The goat's cheese softens the earthy taste of the beetroot to make it quite exceptional.

Ingredients

Serves 3-4

4 medium beetroot
300ml water
1 carton/tin chopped tomatoes
2oz goats cheese
1tsp bouillon
2 cloves of garlic, peeled
Chopped parsley

Method

- Peel and roughly chop beetroot
- Add to the water along with the bouillon and garlic and bring to the boil.
- Simmer for 20 minutes.
- Add the chopped tomatoes and heat through.
- Blend and serve with crumbled goat's cheese and chopped parsley.

MAINS

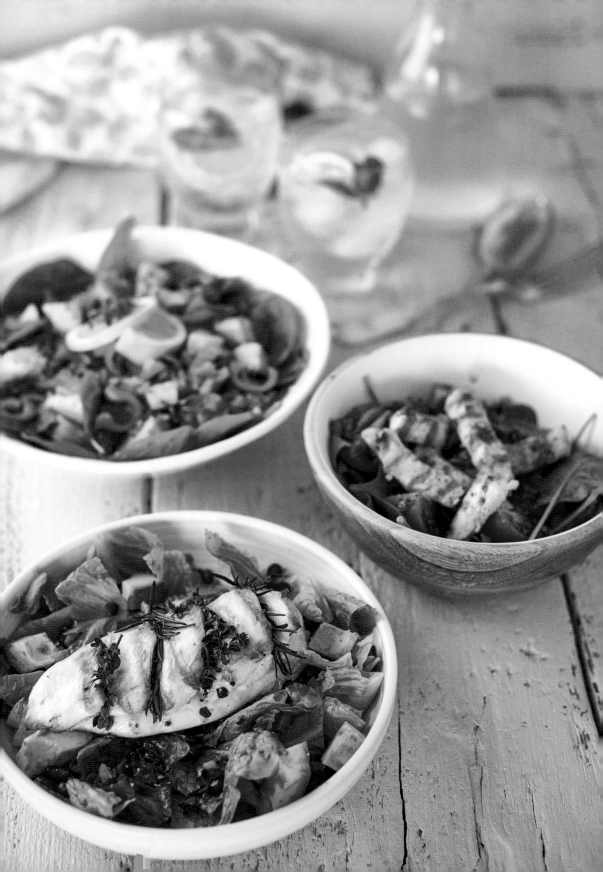

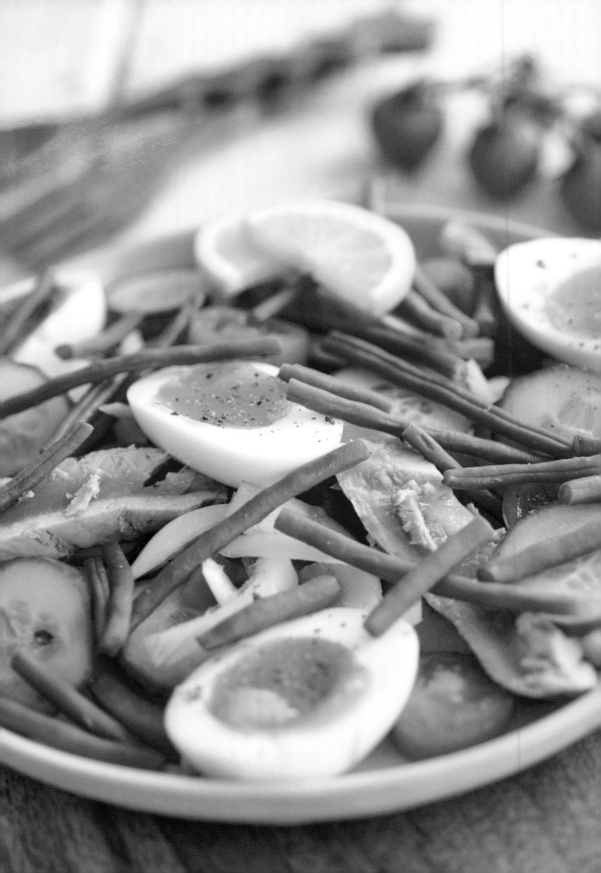

SALAD NIÇOISE

Tuna contains all essential amino acids required by the body for growth and maintenance of lean muscle. It is recommended that you only eat one portion of tuna per week as large fish can potentially contain mercury. For most people, the fish doesn't contain enough mercury to be of concern but it is a consideration for pregnant women, nursing women, babies and young children.

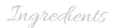

Ingredients

Serves 4

2 tins tuna (or fresh tuna)
4 eggs
1onion
2 red peppers
6 large tomatoes
Half a cucumber
4oz green beans (boiled and cooled)
Mixed herbs
Drizzle of olive oil
2 handfuls of olives

Method

- Boil eggs in water for 7 minutes, before plunging in to ice cold water to prevent over cooking.
- In the meantime, slice tomatoes, cucumber, pepper and onions, then mix in a bowl with the olives.
- Add the tuna and stir in, along with the olive oil.
- Arrange on plates, and then serve with the boiled eggs on top.

PRAWN THAI CURRY

Adding coconut milk to this dish gives a boost of medium chain triglycerides to aid burning of stored fat deposits. It is a delightfully creamy, lightly spiced curry and you can use the base for any protein source that you might have on hand. Turmeric has amazing antioxidant and anti-inflammatory properties to heal and soothe.

Ingredients

Serves 2

400g prawns
1 onion, peeled and sliced
1 red pepper, sliced
3 cloves garlic, peeled and minced
4oz boiled green beans
Half tin coconut milk
1tbsp grape seed oil
Half tsp of each turmeric, coriander
Thai chilli powder and salt to taste

Method

Using a tablespoon of grape seed oil, lightly fry onions and peppers until softened. Add in the green beans, warming through, then remove from the pan.

Fry the prawns and garlic with the spices until they are almost cooked, then add your vegetables back to the pan along with the coconut milk. Heat until warmed through, adjusting the seasoning as desired, then eat immediately.

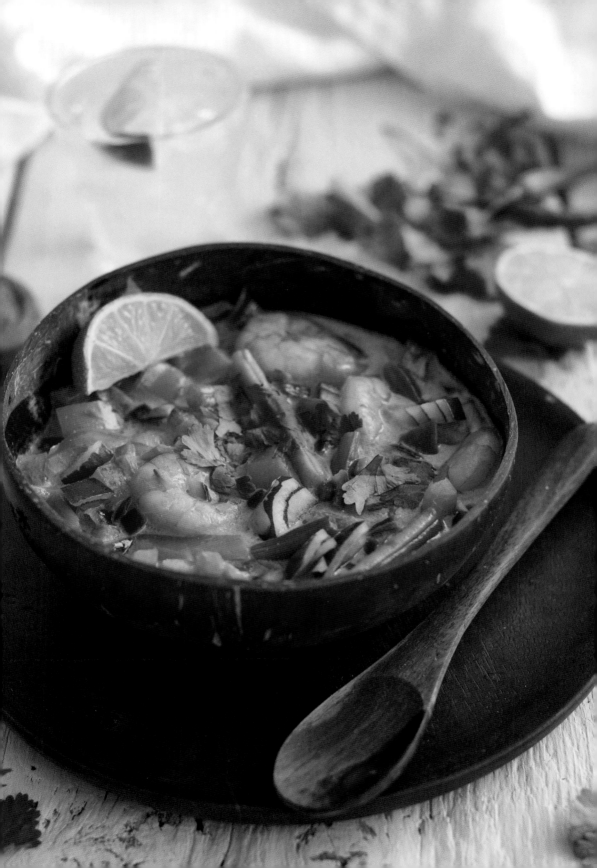

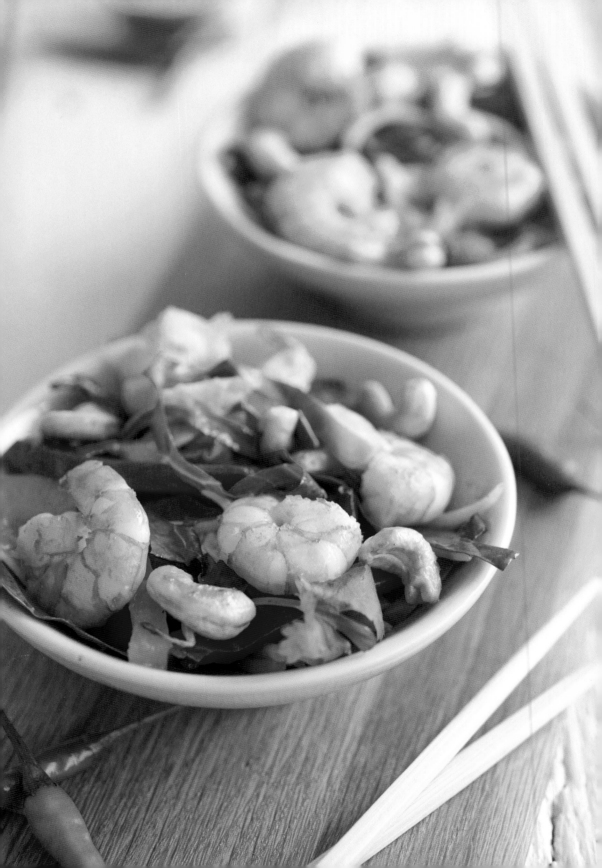

PRAWN & CASHEW STIR FRY

A speedy dish that you can rustle up in a matter of minutes. You could quite literally grab yourself a pack of pre-prepared stir-fry and a pack of prawns on your way home and be eating this within 15 minutes of walking through the door.

Ingredients

Serves 2

400g prawns
1 onion, peeled and sliced
1 red/green pepper, diced
1 large carrot, cut in to thin strips
1 handful mange tout, lightly boiled
1 handful bean sprouts
75g cashew nuts
1 small chilli, de-seeded and finely chopped
1cm cube ginger, finely chopped
3 cloves garlic, finely chopped
Grape seed oil

Method

- Fry the onions gently in grapeseed oil until beginning to soften, then add the peppers, chili and carrots until softened.
- Remove the onion mixture from the pan, then fry the prawns quickly, stirring through the garlic, cashew nuts and ginger.
- Add the vegetables back to the pan, along with the mange tout and bean sprouts, and heat back through. Serve.

TIP
You can vary the protein in all these dishes and substitute for your favourite fish, meat or vegetarian alternative.

Grilled Prawns & Green Salad

Another speedy dish and one that we love on a summer evening. It's reminiscent of Mediterranean holidays.

Ingredients

Serves 2

400g tiger prawns
Grape seed oil, to fry
2 garlic cloves, peeled and minced
Juice of 1 lime
Ground black pepper

For the salad -
Small packet rocket leaves
Handful black olives
1 red pepper, de-seeded and sliced
Small avocado, sliced

Method

• Heat pan or grill, lightly coating with grapeseed oil.
• Cook prawns quickly until starting to go golden.
• Sprinkle with garlic, lime, sea salt and black pepper and continue until fully cooked.
• Arrange on pre-prepared salad.

For the salad –
Prepare just before frying prawns by combining and tossing each of the ingredients together.

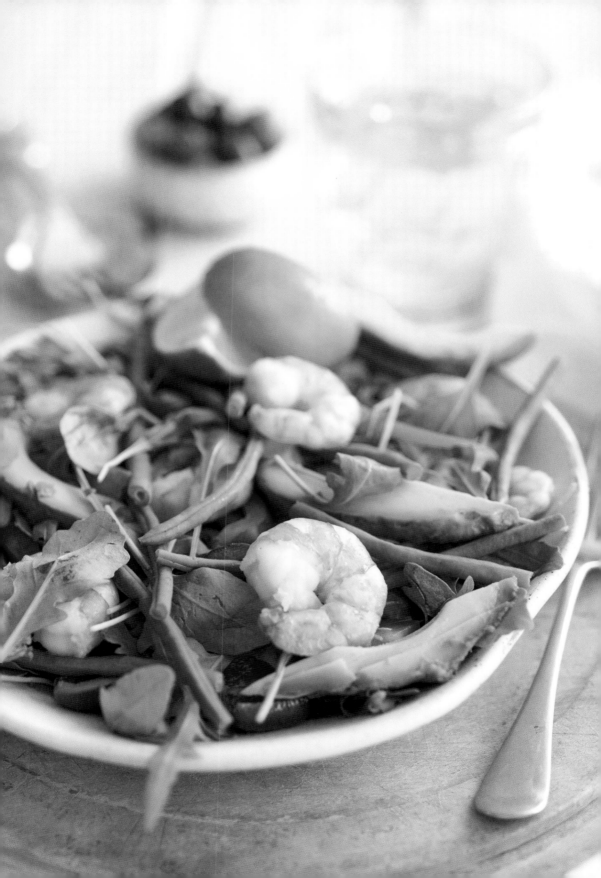

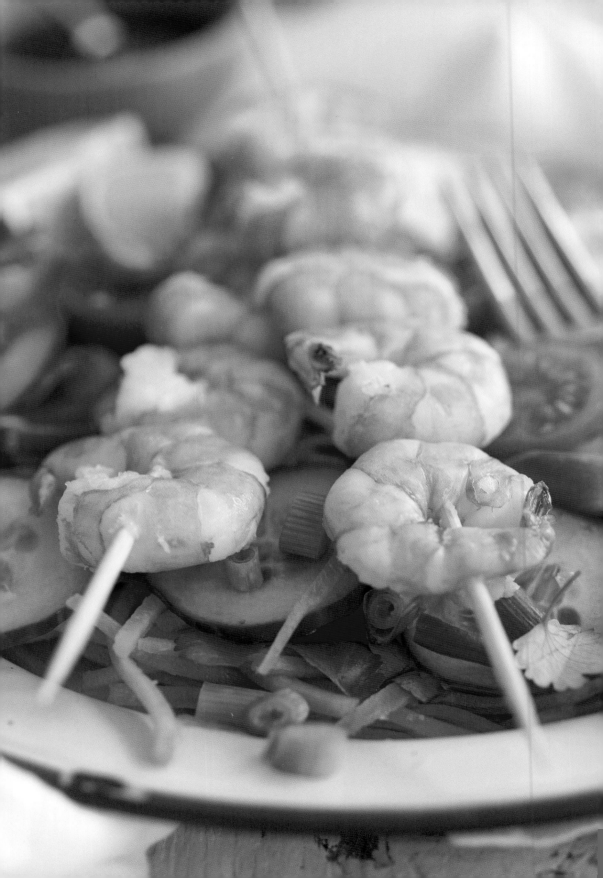

Thai Chicken or Prawn Skewers

Whether it's a Summer BBQ or night in, these skewers are incredibly tasty with healthy fats and fresh vegetables. We've used tamari sauce instead of soy sauce as it is gluten-free and lower in salt.

Ingredients

Serves 2

For the salad -
Half a cucumber
2 carrots
2 cloves garlic, peeled and minced
1cm cube ginger
1 red chili
4 spring onions
Handful boiled green beans
Handful of cherry tomatoes, halved
Juice of 1 lime
6tbsp tamari sauce
2tbsp rice wine vinegar
Handful coriander leaves, chopped

For the skewers:
400g chicken or prawns

Method

- Grate carrots into a bowl.
- Add in the chopped green beans, halved tomatoes and spring onions.
- Crush garlic, chili and ginger and zest of lime, before tipping into the bowl.
- Add in the chopped coriander, along with the splash of rice wine vinegar and tamari sauce, and stir well. Set aside.
- Next, thread chicken cubes or prawns onto skewers and grill or BBQ until cooked through. Serve with pre-prepared salad.

Orange, Avocado & Chicken Salad

You can use leftover chicken or ready-cooked chicken for this recipe. It features our favourite avocado. I love it so much that I could eat it in every meal. Avocado is so nutritious, it's packed with healthy fats, vitamins and minerals and it's a great source of protein.

Ingredients

Serves 1

1 orange, peeled and sliced
Half an avocado, chopped
1 small portion of cooked chicken breast
Handful of spinach leaves
Olive oil, to dress

Method

- Combine ingredients and drizzle with olive oil for a quick lunch.

TIP
Try growing your own salad. The leaves literally pop up in days and most are ready within a month.

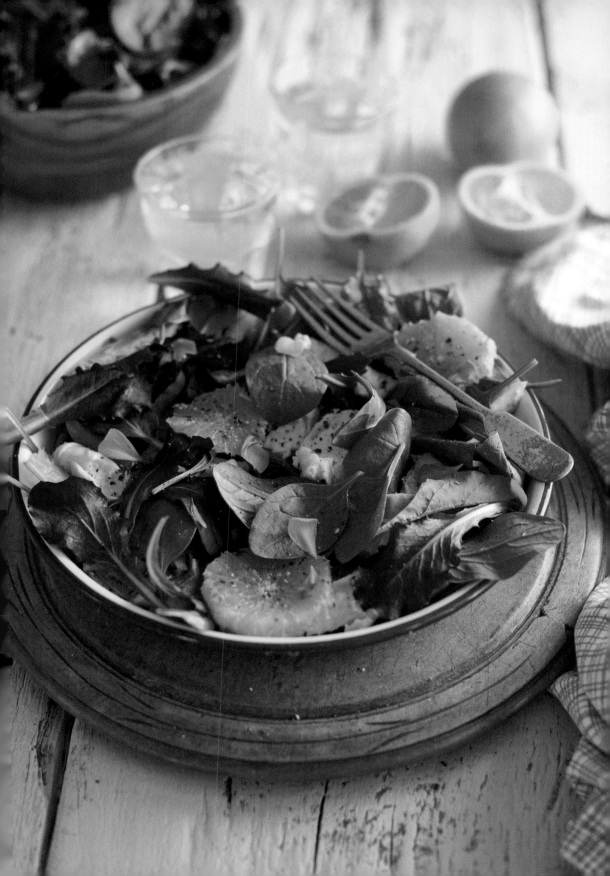

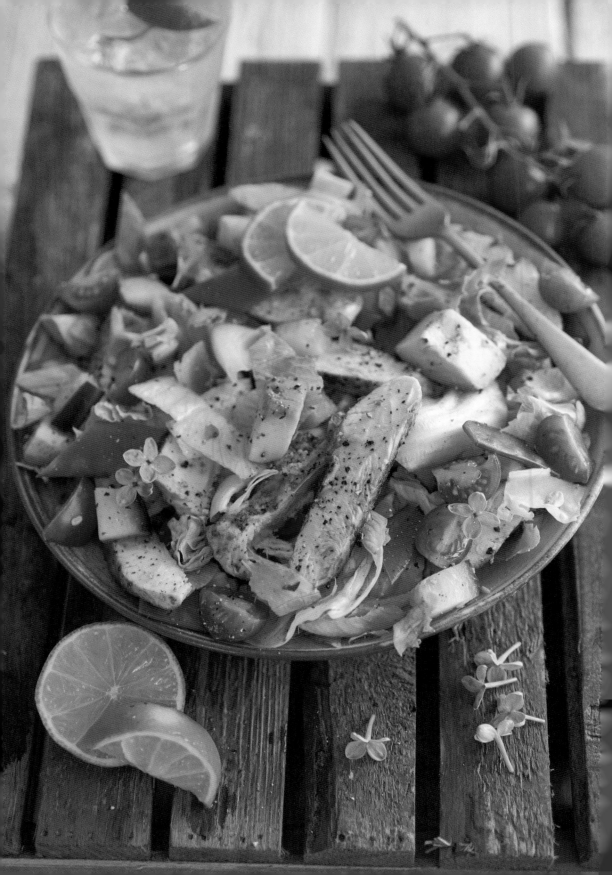

Cajun Chicken with Salad

I first had this dish in New Orleans over 20 years ago. It was an absolute taste sensation to me at the time. The combination of rich Cajun spices blended with cool creamy avocado amazed me and I still love them today.

Ingredients

Serves 2

1 chicken breast per person
1tsp cajun spice mix
1 third of a cucumber, chopped or sliced
4 tomatoes cut into quarters or sliced
Half avocado cut into small cubes
Handful mange tout cut into strips
Half a lettuce
1tbsp grape seed oil

Method

- Bake the chicken in grape seed oil and sprinkle with Cajun spices.
- Arrange the salad whilst the chicken is cooking.
- Once the chicken is cooked, slice and toss through the prepared salad. Enjoy hot or cold.

Easy Herb Chicken

Chicken can sometimes be a little bland on it's own. You might be a little daunted about having to cut into chicken yourself but once you start you will want to try out different herbs and stuffings. The possibilities are endless.

If you are cooking chicken breasts, one of my favourite tips is to make slashes and stuff with fresh sage, parsley or thyme leaves, adding garlic if you wish. If you are cooking a whole bird, you can make slashes in the legs also. Just remember to always cook chicken thoroughly.

Thai Prawns

Prawns are a good source of unsaturated fat, which makes up the majority of its fat content. Unsaturated fats can help to improve your blood cholesterol levels when you eat them instead of saturated or transfats. They are also a good source of Omega-3 fatty acids, calcium, potassium, phosphorous and Vitamins A and E. They are though quite high in sodium. This recipe is a healthy option to having a takeaway curry and has all the taste.

Ingredients

Serves 2

400g prawns
2tbsp grape seed oil
Half a lemon, or for more zing half lime
2 cloves chopped garlic
1cm cubed chopped ginger
Chili pepper (optional)
Parsley

Method

• Marinade prawns in the above ingredients for 30 minutes. Next, lightly fry the marinated prawns until cooked through, before serving with a super vitamin salad or gently-simmered dark green vegetables.

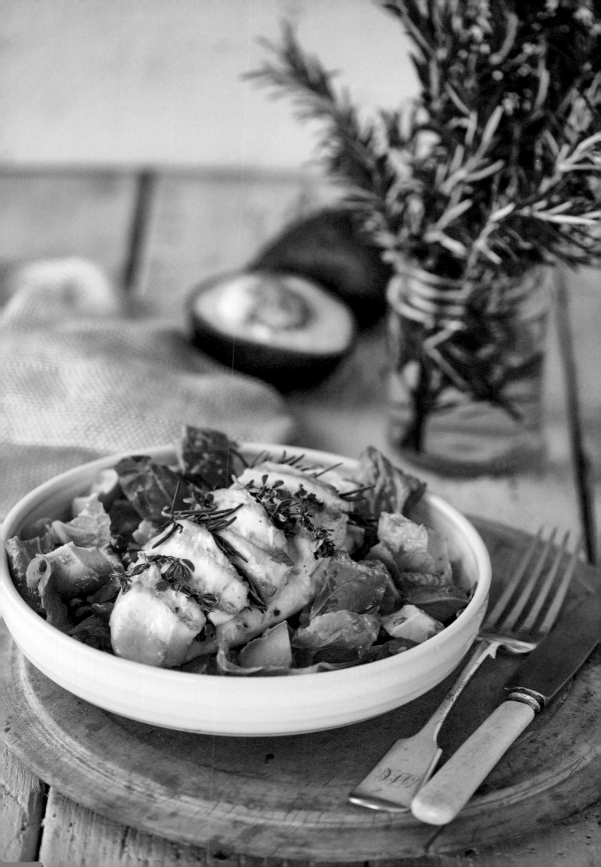

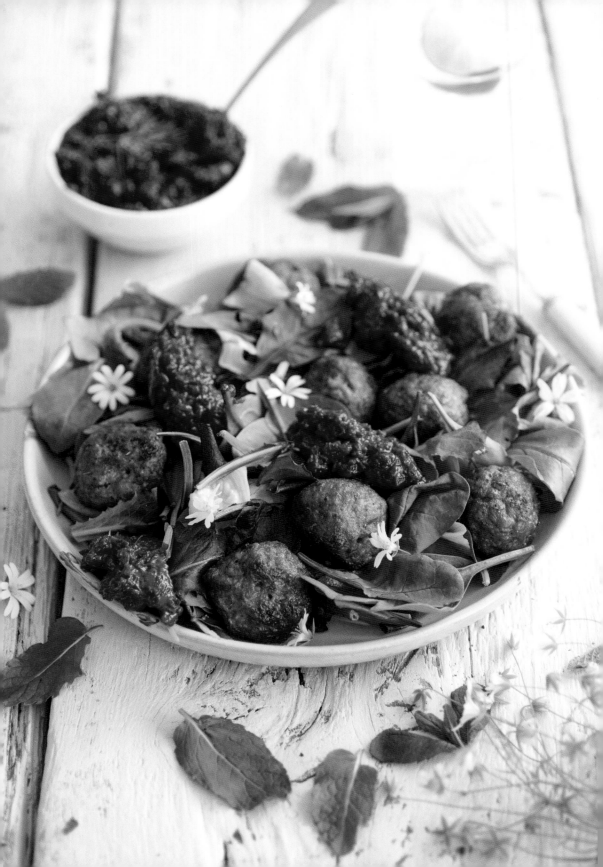

LAMB MEATBALLS WITH BEETROOT DIP & GREEN SALAD

If you crave for a burger then this is a great alternative to having a large bun with fries. You can use any ground meat for the recipe. Those with Blood Type O tend to fare better with some red meat in our diets. Blood Type O ancestors were meat eaters and our constitution is more suited to it than other blood types. Dietary patterns are changing and more people are choosing to be vegetarian or vegan but you may find that adding some lean meat might be beneficial.

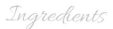

For the meatballs -

150g of lean minced lamb per person (beef or turkey would do)
Half a small onion, finely chopped (allow half onion per person)
Sprinkle of dried mint
Salt and pepper

- Combine the meatball ingredients and form in to flat balls. Fry gently on both sides until cooked through, then serve with the beetroot dip* and green salad.

see beetroot dip recipe in dips and dressings on page 154

Quinoa & Roast Vegetables

Quinoa is gluten-free and high in protein, it has almost twice as much fibre as most other grains. One of the most nutrient-dense grains, it contains iron, lysine, magnesium, Vitamin B2 and manganese. Quinoa is so easy to cook and you can prepare it in bulk to add to dishes throughout the week.

Ingredients

Serves 2

1½ cups quinoa
4 spring onions, diced
1 courgette, peeled and chopped
Half a red pepper, deseeded and chopped
1 clove garlic, peeled and minced
1 dessert spoon olive oil

Method

- Pre-heat the oven to 180C.
- Quinoa is a delightful nutty tasting seed and can be used instead of couscous. To prepare, add the quinoa to three cups of water and cook on a low heat until light and fluffy (around 20 minutes).
- In the meantime, chop the spring onions and put on one side. Prepare the roast vegetables by popping peppers and courgettes in to pre-heated oven for 20 minutes.
- Add olive oil, chopped raw spring onions and parsley with finely chopped garlic to the quinoa.
- Once the roast vegetables are cooked, stir in to the quinoa and dish up.

TIP
If desired you can add the juice of half a lime and sprinkle with coriander.

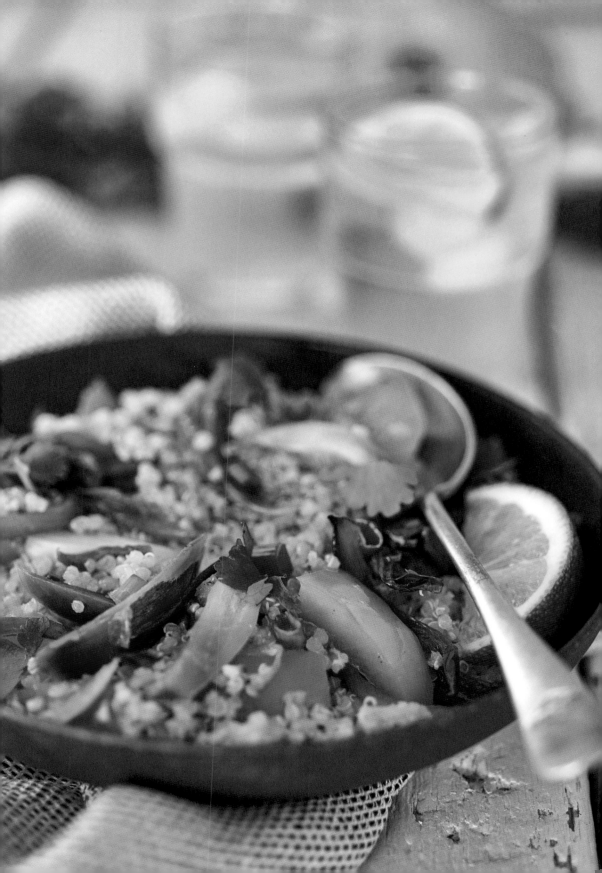

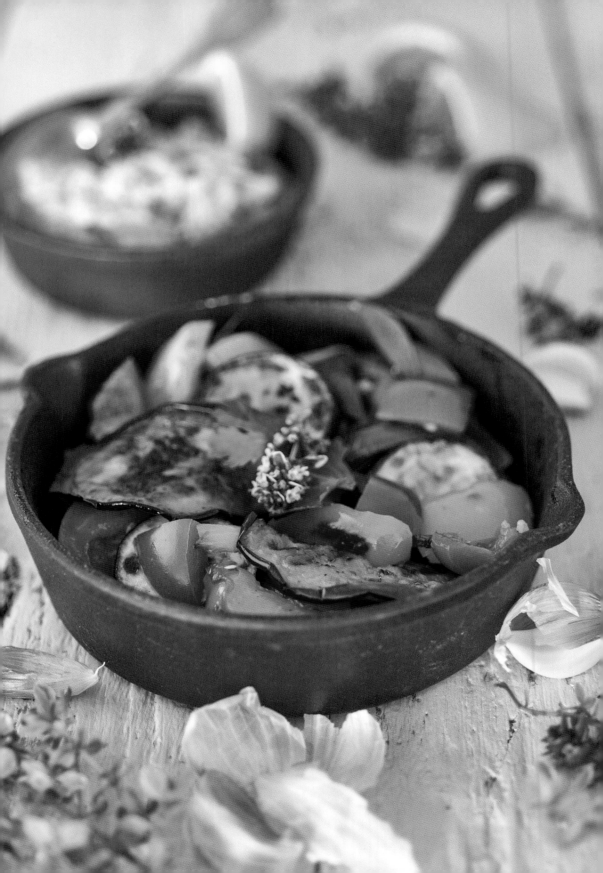

MEDITERRANEAN VEGETABLES WITH BEAN MASH

  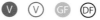

We love this dish, whether we're sitting out on a hot summer's night in Spain or around the stove in winter back in the UK. Hope it might become one of your favourites too.

Ingredients

Serves 2

1 pepper, deseeded and sliced
1 aubergine, sliced
2 courgettes. sliced
2tbsp olive oil

For the mash -
One can of cannelini drained and rinsed
100ml stock
One clove garlic, crushed
1tbsp chopped coriander
Lemon wedges to serve

Method

- Gently fry the vegetables in oil until softened.
- In the meantime, heat the beans in a saucepan with the stock until heated through, before mashing and stirring in the coriander.
- Divide portions of the mash into two bowls, then top with the vegetables and serve with lemon.

TIP
You can add whatever vegetables you have in the fridge for variation.

Pearl Barley & Mushroom Supper

Pearl barley is a lovely healthy alternative for traditional risotto rice, it provides minerals, fibre, selenium, copper, chromium and magnesium. It's a wonderfully versatile grain with a rich nutty flavour and can be used in most dishes where you would normally have rice.

Ingredients

Serves 2

120g pearl barley
500ml water
Half tsp bouillon
1 onion, peeled and finely chopped
500g chestnut mushrooms, quartered
2 cloves garlic, finely chopped
Small bunch parsley, finely chopped
Olive oil
Salt and pepper, to taste

Method

- Add the pearl barley and bouillon to the water and bring to a boil, turning down to simmer for 30-40 minutes, or until softened and all liquid is absorbed.
- Next, gently fry the onions in the olive oil until softened.
- In separate pan, fry the mushrooms and garlic until softened.
- To serve, toss together the cooked pearl barley with the onion and mushroom mixtures, then stir in the parsley. Enjoy.

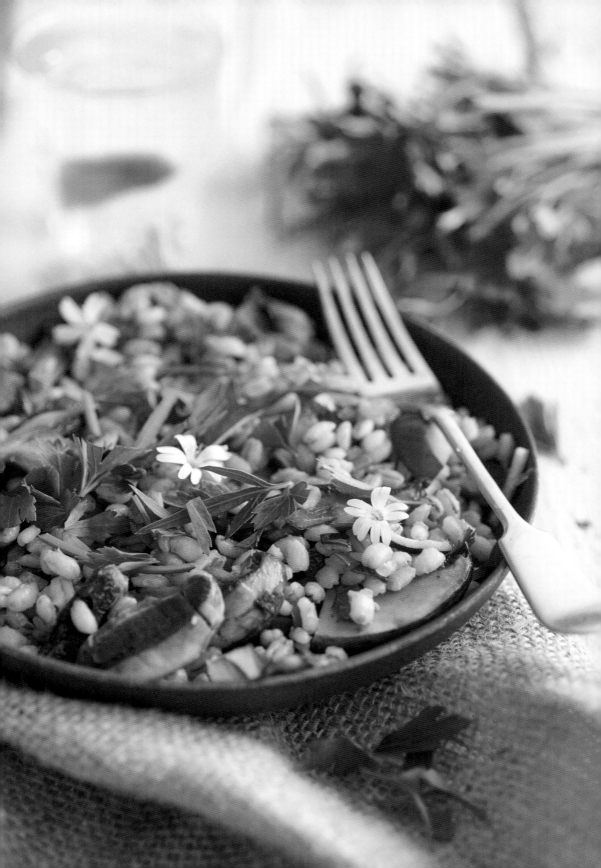

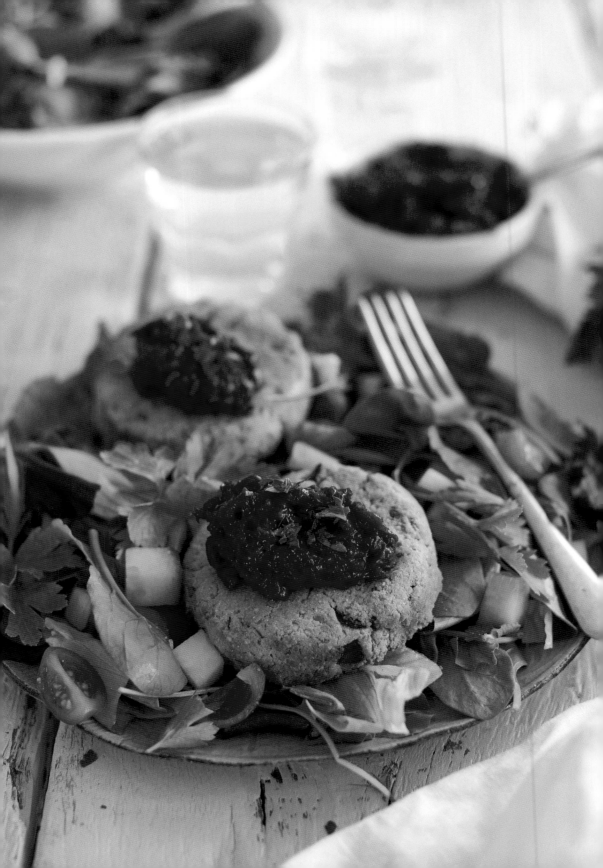

CHICKPEA BURGERS

Chickpeas are considered to be a vegetable and protein food, helping you to hit two important nutrient food groups at once. They have a nutty flavour and can be used whole or blended into pâtés and dips.

Ingredients

Makes 4 burgers

1 (15.5oz) can of chickpeas, drained and rinsed
Half cup chopped red onion
Half cup chopped fresh parsley
1tbsp fresh lemon juice
1tsp ground cumin
1tsp ground coriander
Half tsp salt
2 garlic cloves, peeled and minced

Method

- Blend the chickpeas until smooth, then combine with the remaining ingredients and shape into patties.
- Shallow fry until cooked.
- Serve with salad of your choice.

ROAST AUBERGINE, SAUTÉED ONIONS, CHOPPED WALNUTS & POMEGRANATE

Aubergines are often an overlooked vegetable low in calories but rich in vitamins and minerals. They contain chlorogenic acid a compound known for its high antioxidant activity and which can lower cholesterol levels.

Ingredients

Serves 2

2 aubergines
75g walnuts
Half a pomegranate
Sprig of parsley leaves, shredded
1 large onion

Method

- Grill slices of the aubergine and gently sauté slices of onion.
- To serve, top the aubergine with the sautéed onions, then sprinkle with pomegranate, walnuts and a scattering of fresh mint leaves.

TIP
You can vary this recipe by adding creamy soft goat's cheese.

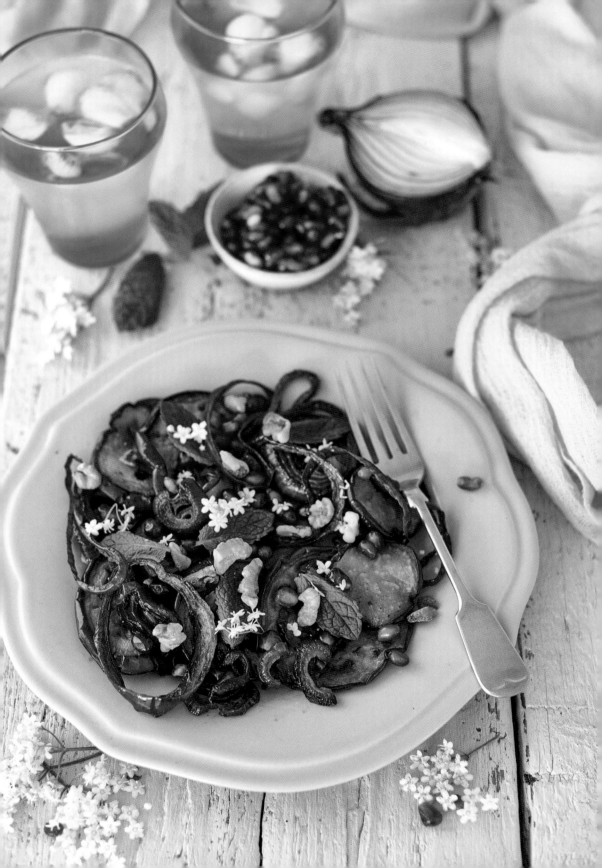

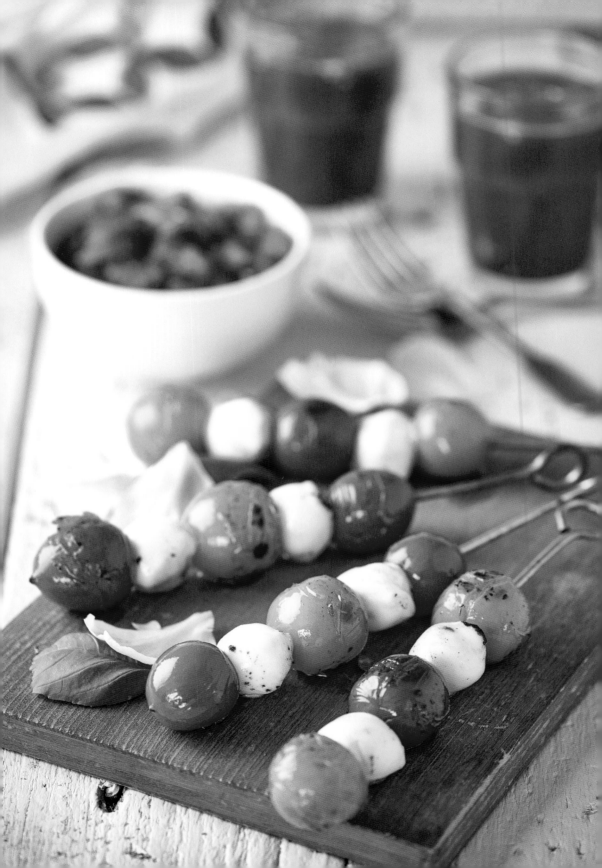

Mozzarella Kebabs

Ingredients

Serves 2

12 cherry tomatoes
12 mozzarella balls
Basil
Oil

Method

Thread tomatoes and mozzarella onto sticks, then drizzle with oil and grill gently until browned and the mozzarella is gooey. Serve with sprigs of basil.

Alfredo's Salad

This is such a gorgeous salad. It's the house salad at a small Spanish restaurant in San Pedro, on the Costa del Sol. The salad in the restaurant has changed over the years but our version remains as we remember it. The boys have it alongside their starter but it would do me for the whole meal.

Ingredients

Serves 4 as a starter or 2 as a main dish

Half a lettuce
1 tin tuna, drained
2 hard-boiled eggs, cut into quarters

For the salad -
6 salad tomatoes, sliced
Half a cucumber, sliced
1 red pepper, deseeded and sliced
1 onion, peeled and sliced
One grated carrot
Finely sliced beetroot
Handful back olives

Method

• Toss together the salad ingredients in a bowl.
• Arrange on a bed of lettuce.
• Top with the tuna and eggs, then serve and enjoy.

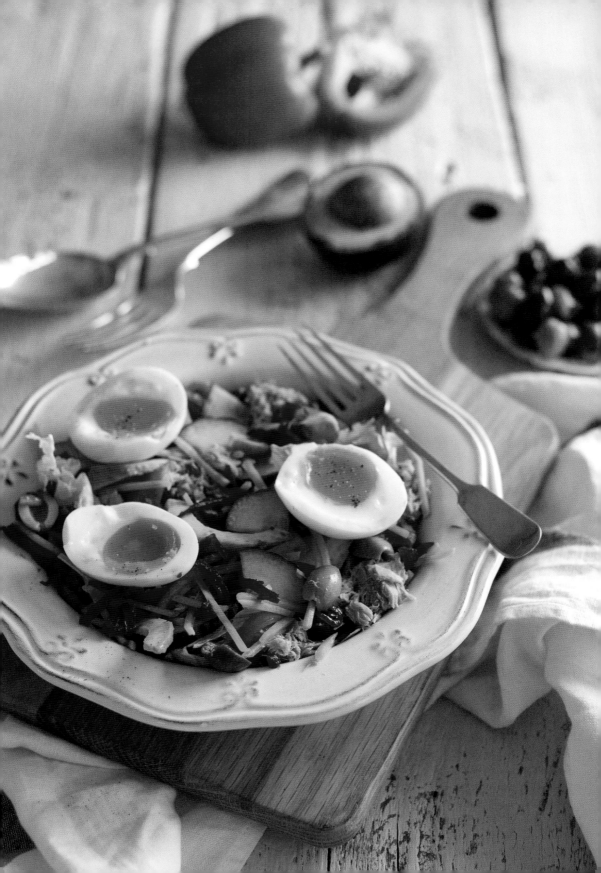

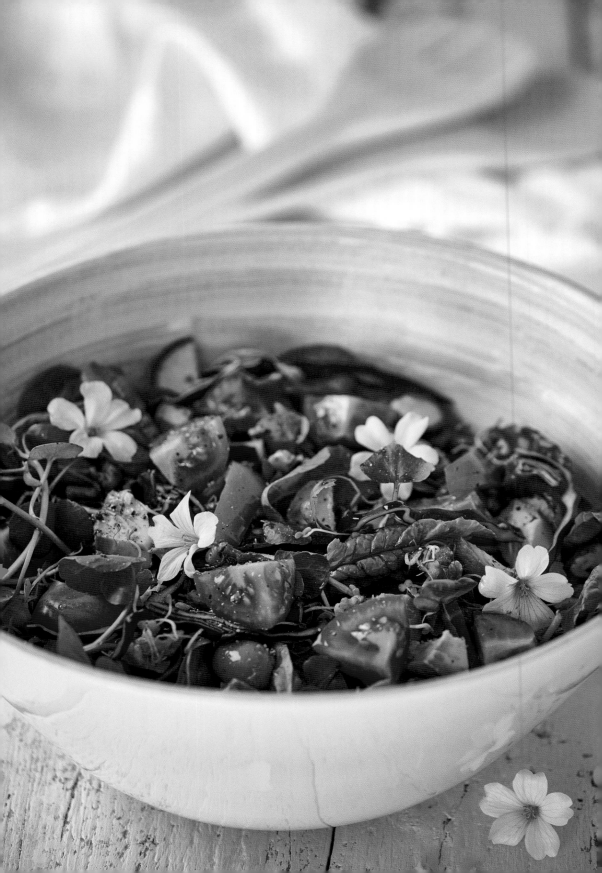

Rejuvenated Salad

This salad is packed with amazing nutrients, vitamins, minerals, antioxidants, proteins and essential fatty acids. We've combined supercharged nutrition in a bowl to nourish and enjoy.

Ingredients

Serves 4

Large handful of spinach or Swiss chard
Bag of watercress or alternate green leaves
Half a red cabbage, finely sliced
1 red pepper, deseeded and chopped
1 red onion chopped
Half a cucumber, sliced or cubed
6 salad tomatoes, sliced or quartered
Handful olives
1 avocado chopped
Alfalfa sprouts, to top (if available)
10 walnuts, broken and sprinkled
Pumpkin or sunflower seeds, to sprinkle

Method

• Wash each of the salad ingredients and chop onions, tomato and cucumber.
• Peel and scoop out flesh of avocado.
• Combine the ingredients, topping with alfalfa sprouts and sprinkling with sunflower or pumpkin seeds.

Super Green Quinoa Salad with Avocado Dressing

Supercharged goodness with protein rich quinoa and a creamy smooth avocado dressing.

Ingredients

Serves 2

250g quinoa
500ml boiling water (add a teaspoon of
vegetable bouillon)
1 chopped avocado
1 red pepper, deseeded and chopped
Half a chopped cucumber
Handful fresh coriander
8 cherry tomatoes
Juice of half lime

Method

• Add quinoa to the boiling water, along
  with the bouillon
• Turn down the heat and simmer for 15-20
  minutes until softened and all the water
  has been absorbed.
• Drain quinoa, then toss in the vegetables
  before stirring in the lime juice.
• Top with fresh, finely-chopped coriander.

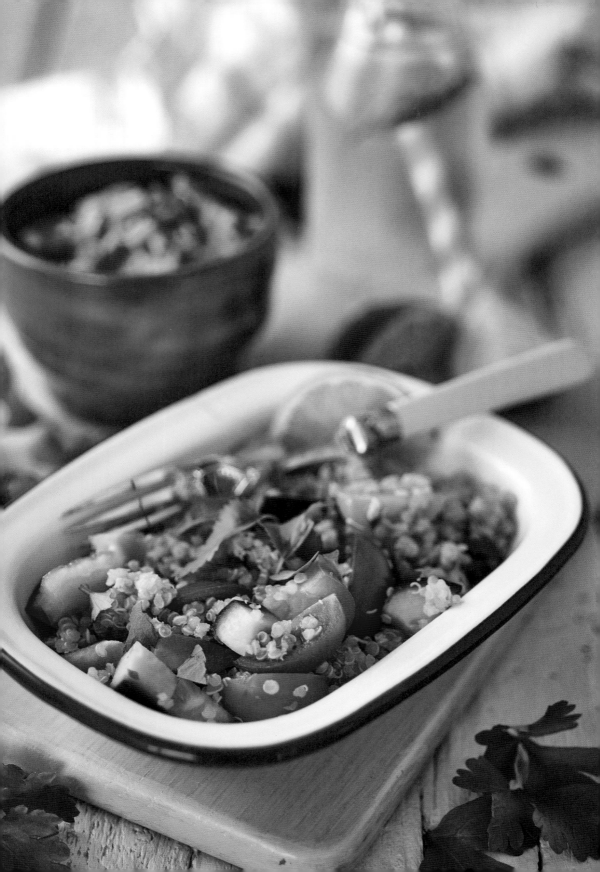

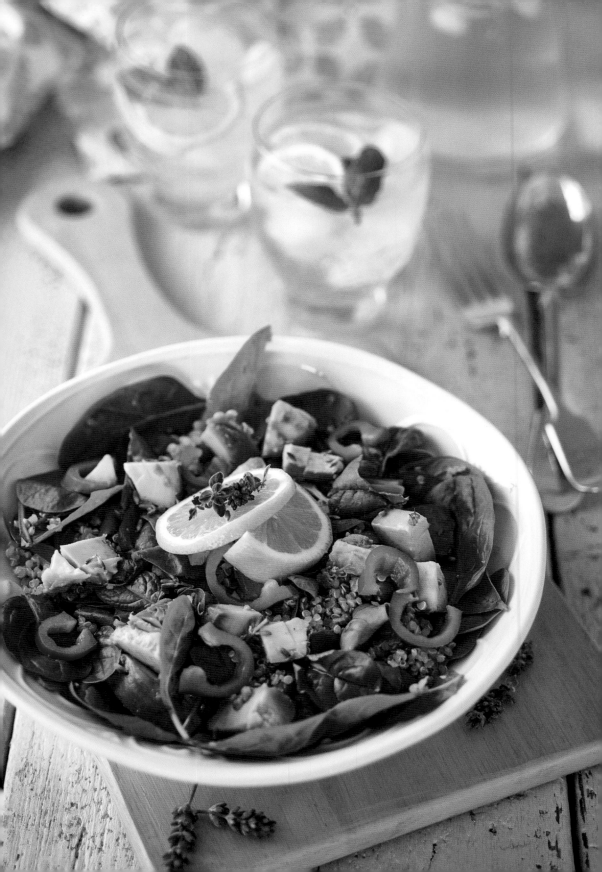

Super Green Quinoa Salad

Ingredients

Serves 2

250g quinoa
500ml boiling water (add a teaspoon of vegetable bouillon)
1 onion, peeled and chopped
1 pack Swiss chard, chopped
1 pack spinach
Quarter of a red pepper
100g frozen peas
2 cloves garlic, finely chopped
Half a lemon, juiced.

Method

- Add quinoa to boiling water along with the bouillon.
- Turn down the heat and simmer for 15-20 minutes, cooking until softened and all the water has been absorbed.
- Meanwhile prepare and chop up vegetables and stir-fry them gently, adding in the garlic just before they are fully cooked.
- Drain the quinoa, toss in the vegetables, and then drizzle over the juice of half a lemon.

WARM KALE & SPINACH SALAD WITH AVOCADO

Not everyone can tolerate kale as it is very high in fibre and some sugars. Kale is a cruciferous vegetable in the same family as cabbage: it contains fructans and galactans which can be hard to digest. It also has raffinose which is composed of several sugar molecules, which is also hard to break down and can ferment in the colon, causing bloating and abdominal pain. Cooking the leaves lightly can soften the fibres to make them more digestible. But if you suffer from Irritable bowel syndrome, then kale is best left alone.

Ingredients

Serves 2

125g spinach leaves
Bunch of kale,washed and patted dry
Half an avocado, chopped
Dressing of choice
Pine nuts
Himalayan salt, according to taste

Method

- Gently stir fry the kale and add spinach leaves to slightly wilt them.
- In the meantime, mix up and prepare dressing.
- Toss together the spinach, kale and avocado, then drizzle over dressing.
- Top with pine nuts.

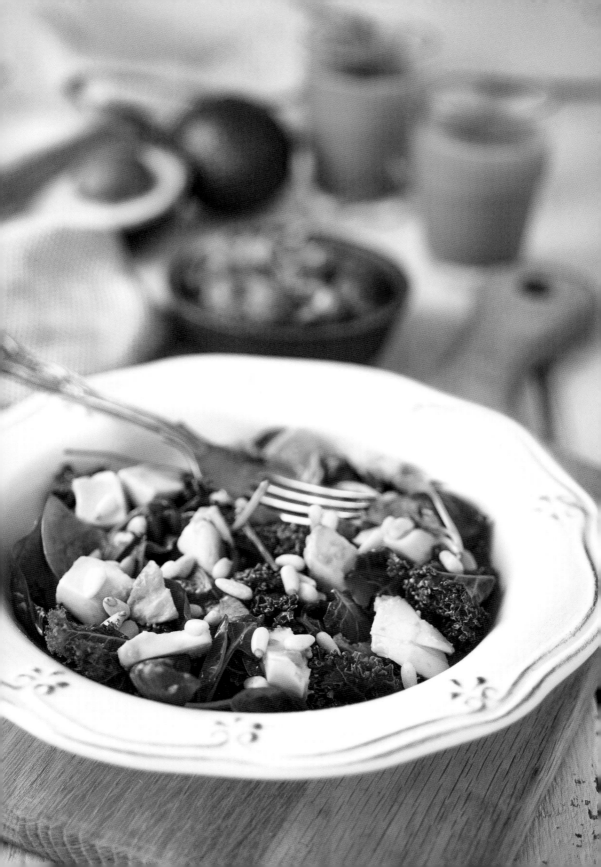

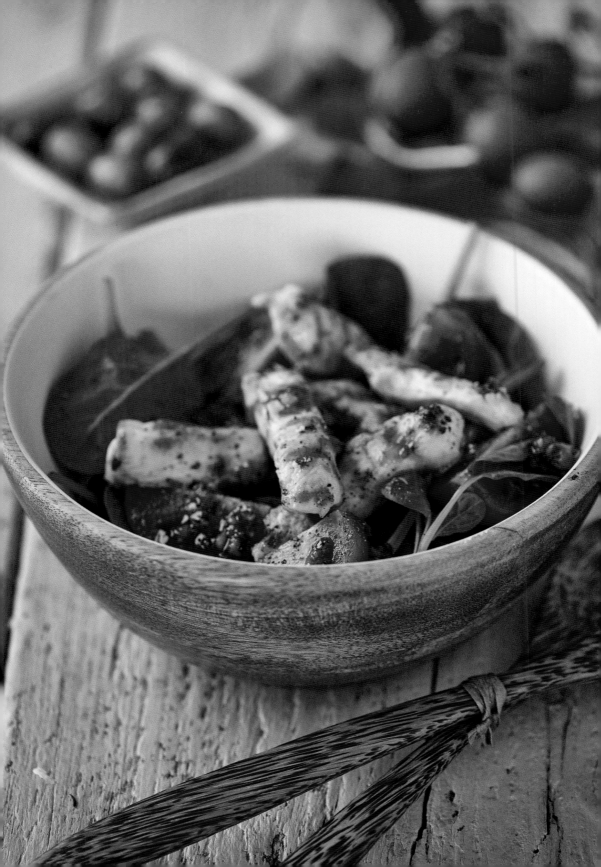

Chicken & Spinach Salad

This has to be the quickest salad to make and so easy to prepare if you are short on time.

Ingredients

Serves 2

2 breasts cooked chicken
Handful of spinach
4 tomatoes
6 olives
Drizzle over with olive oil or one of the dressings from page 149

Method

Simply toss together the cooked chicken, spinach, tomatoes and olives, then drizzle over your dressing of choice.

GREEK SALAD

Who doesn't love a traditional Greek salad made with fresh leaves and vegetables? it's a great starter or served as a main course.

Ingredients

Serves 2

125g spinach
Half a lettuce
4 cherry tomatoes
200g feta cheese
6 black olives
Half a red onion
Half a small cucumber
Fresh mint, finely chopped
Olive oil

Method

• Chop lettuce and mix with the spinach.
• Halve the tomatoes and chop the feta.
• Slice onions and cucumber, then combine your veggies and toss with the mint.
• Drizzle with olive oil and serve.

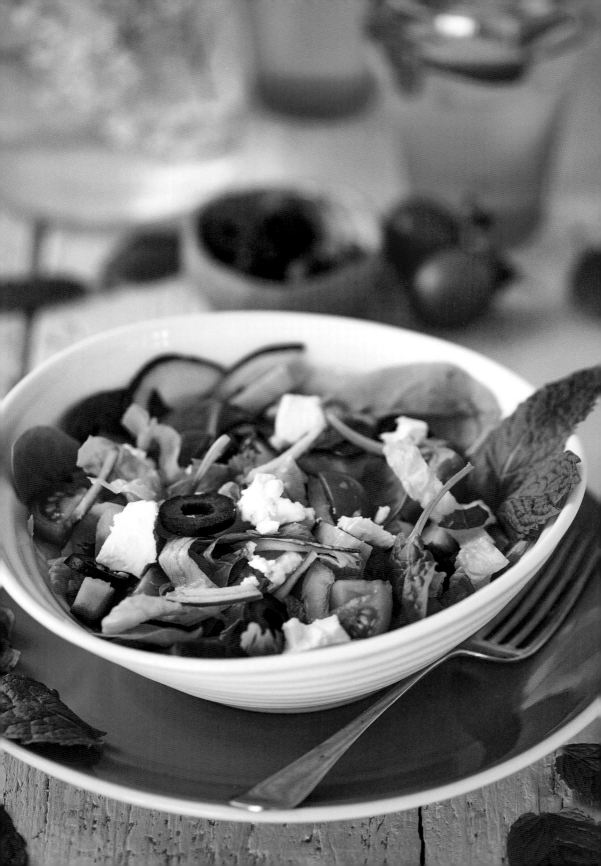

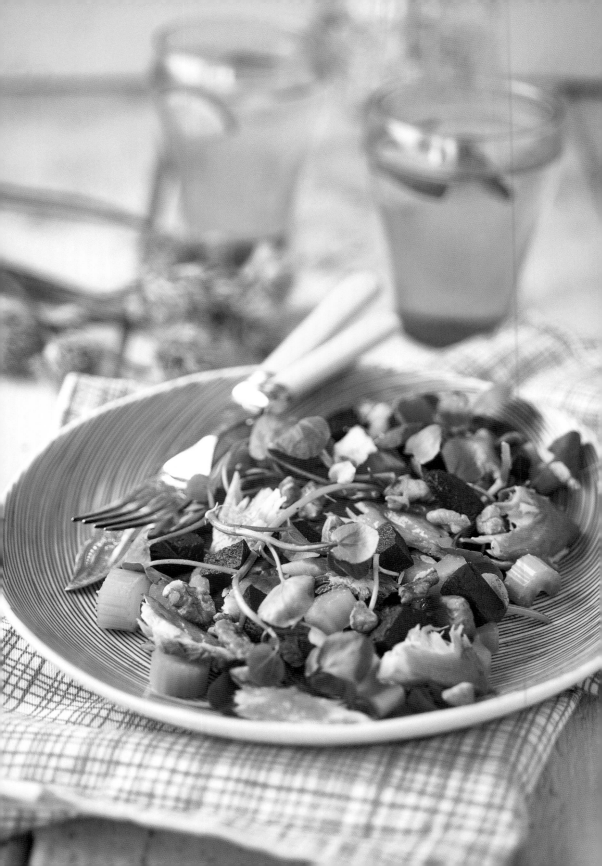

MACKEREL & BEETROOT SALAD

Get your fill of Omega-3 with any oily fish. Mackerel is so reasonable in the shops too. Then vamp up a traditional coleslaw by adding some super nutritious veggies with a few brain-boosting walnuts.

Ingredients

Serves 2

2 - 3 cooked mackerel fillets
2 small beetroot, chopped
4 sticks celery, chopped
75g walnuts
100g watercress
125g spinach
Salad dressing *or* olive oil, mixed with
lemon and garlic to taste

Method

• Arrange the watercress and spinach bowl.
• Add in the chopped celery, beetroot, walnuts and mackerel.
• Finish with dressing.

Ratatouille
(excellent with fish)

Another Mediterranean staple dish, originating from the Nice area of France. Originally the dish was just courgettes, tomatoes, red and green peppers, onions and garlic but nowadays aubergine is usually added to the list of ingredients. The dish is rich in carotenoids due to the highly-pigmented peppers and tomatoes, making it full of health-giving antioxidants.

Ingredients

Serves 2

2tbsp grape seed oil
250g courgettes, sliced
1 medium onion, finely chopped
200g ripe tomatoes or tinned tomatoes
1 garlic clove, chopped
Chilli flakes or cayenne pepper
(optional)
Fresh herbs of choice
You can also add any other vegetable to this dish - peppers, aubergine and mushrooms are all good.

Method

- Add oil to a frying pan and heat.
- Tip in the onions, chili and garlic and fry gently until onion is golden. Set aside.
- If using fresh tomatoes, place in a bowl and pour over boiling water. Prick their skins with a sharp knife, then leave for a minute and drain. Peel and chop.
- Next, fry courgettes gently, then add all the other ingredients including peeled, chopped tomatoes (or tinned tomatoes).
- Heat through, then season to taste and top with fresh herbs of your choice.

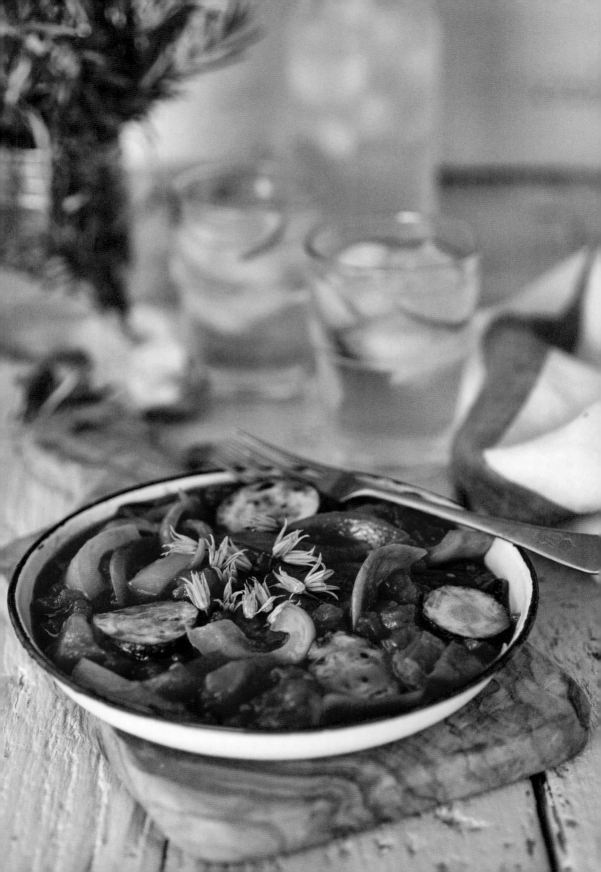

DIPS & DRESSINGS

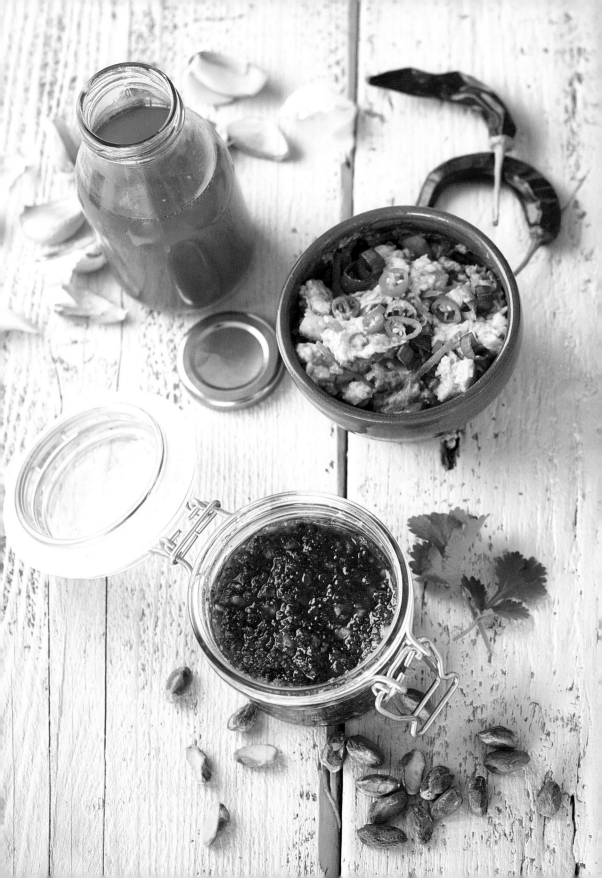

Avocado Dressing

This is a gorgeous dip or stir into salads as a thick creamy dressing. It's actually delicious stirred into quinoa or you can thin it down with yogurt or olive oil to make a runnier dressing.

Ingredients

1 avocado
1 clove garlic, minced
1tbsp tahini
2 chopped spring onions
Dash of chili powder
Small amount salt, to taste

Method

- Mash avocado
- Stir in minced garlic, tahini, chili and add spring onions.
- Season with salt to taste.

Tomato & Red Pepper Salsa

A spicy salsa which complements fish or sweet potatoes perfectly.

Ingredients

1 tin of chopped tomatoes
1 red pepper, deseeded and sliced
1 red onion, peeled and finely chopped
2 cloves garlic, finely chopped
Sprig of basil, shredded

Method

Fry onion and pepper in hot oil until softened, then add the garlic and cook until golden. Add the tomatoes and cook until heated through, stirring through the basil. Enjoy warm, or leave to cool and serve as a dip.

Mustard & Olive Oil Dressing

Ingredients

200ml olive oil
Juice half lemon
2 cloves garlic grated
Salt and pepper to taste
Optional:
Add 1tsp of Dijon mustard for an alternative flavour

Method

Simply stir together the ingredients until smooth, tasting and adjusting as desired.

Basic Salad Dressing

If you don't have time to make this up you can always go with a shop-bought version but try to avoid ones that are high in sugar.

Ingredients

1 cup olive oil
Half cup walnut oil
1 clove garlic, crushed
1 small red chilli, deseeded and chopped
Juice of half a lemon
Pinch salt and pepper

Method

Whizz together the ingredients until smooth. Pour into an airtight container or jam jar, or serve immediately drizzled over your favourite salad.

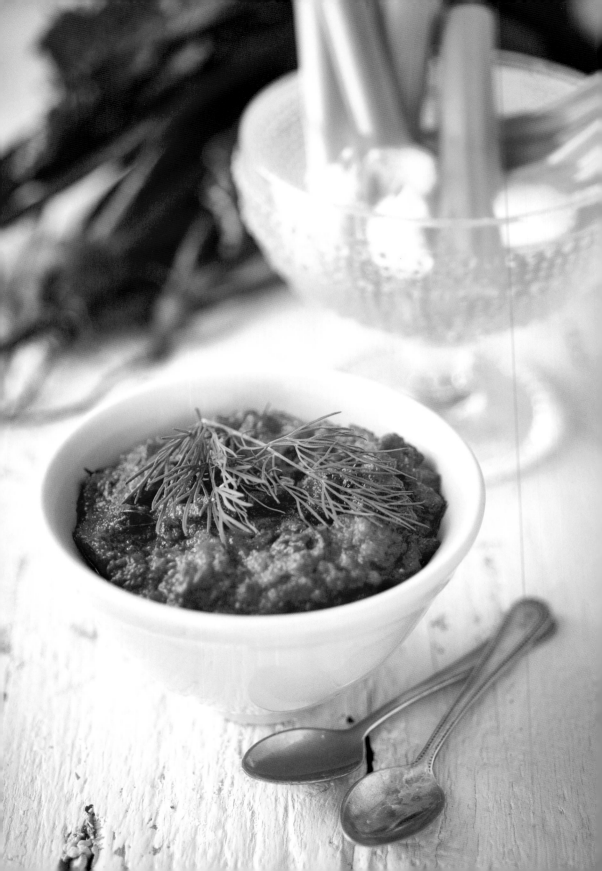

BEETROOT DIP

A lovely dip to get the goodness from this earthy vegetable. Just be sure that you prepare in a pot bowl rather than plastic as the deep rich pigments of beetroot will stain a plastic bowl or pot.

Ingredients

2 medium cooked beetroots
Half onion, chopped
1 clove garlic
200g Greek yogurt
Chopped dill
2tsp olive oil

Method

- Mash beetroot with a fork until almost smooth.
- Stir in the olive oil, along with the finely-chopped garlic and onions, and then mix in the yogurt.
- Add salt and pepper to flavor, then stir in the dill. Serve immediately, or place in the fridge in an airtight container to cool and serve later.

PISTACHIO PESTO

A different version of pesto for you to try. The ones in the supermarket are normally made from basil or peppers. You can actually use most leaves and nuts to create a whole range of different flavours. I even made one out of carrot leaves once and it was lovely so try to be creative and we'd love to see what you come up with.

Ingredients

150g shelled pistachios
1 cup fresh coriander
75ml olive oil
2 cloves chopped garlic
3tbsp Parmesan

Method

Blend all ingredients until you have desired texture. Stir in an airtight container, or serve immediately.

Drinks

Turmeric Latte

A deliciously warming drink with health boosting turmeric, ginger and cinnamon. You can use any milk - we used coconut for ours but try almond milk or organic dairy milk.

Ingredients

Serves 2

350ml warmed coconut milk
1tsp each of turmeric, ginger, cinnamon, coconut nectar
Pinch black pepper

Method

- Blend ingredients until smooth and top with a sprinkle of cinnamon. Take care if milk is very hot.
- Pour into mugs and enjoy immediately.

Beetroot Latte

This is a great drink to give you energy throughout the day. Beetroot gently dilates the arteries to allow the blood to flow more efficiently, while beetroot powders are used by athletes to increase their endurance.

Ingredients

Serves 2

350ml warmed almond milk
1tsp beetroot powder
1tsp coconut nectar

Method

- Blend ingredients until smooth and top with a sprinkle of cinnamon. Take care if milk is very hot.
- Pour into mugs and enjoy immediately.

Matcha Latte

Matcha is the king of green teas. It is thought to have many times more antioxidants than regular green tea. We made ours up into a smooth latte but you can add it to water if you prefer.

Ingredients

Serves 2

350ml warmed coconut milk
1tsp matcha powder
1tsp coconut nectar

Method

- Blend ingredients until smooth and top with a sprinkle of cinnamon. Take care if milk is very hot.
- Pour into mugs and enjoy immediately.

Spiced Chili Cacao

This is a rich warming combination. South Americans have put these ingredients together for centuries but we are only just discovering it. Now that we have, it's definitely one to keep on our list.

Ingredients

Serves 2

350ml almond milk
One small red chili cut in half with seeds removed – leave the stalk on
2tsp ground cacao
1tsp coconut nectar or honey

Method

Add a tablespoon of milk and one teaspoon ground cacao to each cup and blend together into a paste.

Heat rest of almond milk with chili. Once warm, remove the chili and blend the milk and cacao together, taking care if hot.

Add a teaspoon of nectar or honey.

Avocado Smoothie

I was amazed how delicious this smoothie is. It took a while to convince me to try avocado blended into a drink but it really is very lovely.

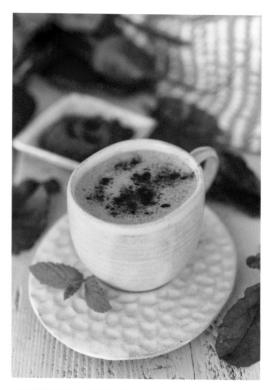

Ingredients

Serves 2

250g spinach
1 kiwi
Half a cucumber
1 ripe avocado
Squeeze of fresh lime
Water as needed

Method

- Juice the spinach, kiwi and half a cucumber
- Blend with the avocado until smooth, adding a little water if necessary to help the blending process. Add a squeeze of lime, blending once more to combine, then pour into glasses and drink immediately.

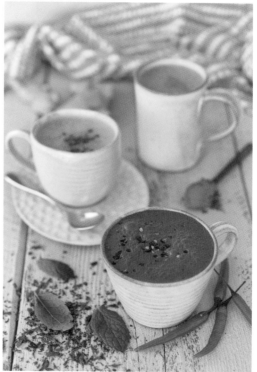

Dedicated to our children Ben, Lois, Lucy, Julia and Russ who've endured testing all our products from concept to production.

Thank you and love you all so much.

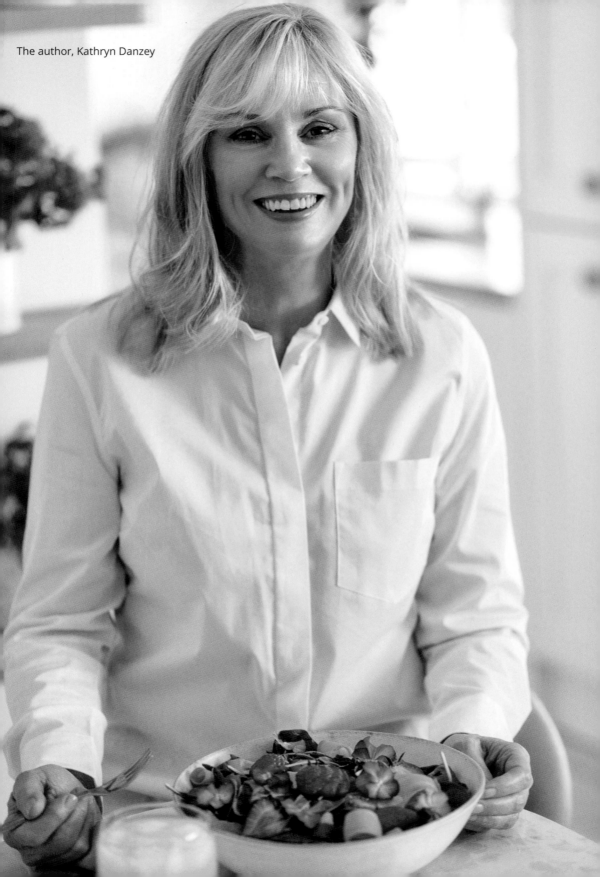

The author, Kathryn Danzey